Jan Abas

Computers in
Health and Fitness

Studentlitteratur Chartwell-Bratt

© Jan Abas and Chartwell Bratt Ltd, 1988

Chartwell-Bratt (Publishing and Training) Ltd
ISBN 0-86238-155-X

Printed in Sweden,
Studentlitteratur, Lund

ISBN 91-44-28201-X   1   2   3   4   5   6   7   8   9   10 | 1992 91 90 89 88

Contents

Acknowledgements

I would like to thank all those who helped me in the writing of this book. Many grateful thanks to:

Mr. John Hornsby and Dr. John Mathews of the University College of North Wales Bangor, Dr. Barry Wyatt of the Institute of Terrestrial Ecology, Bangor and Dr. Peter Smith of Ysbyty Gwynedd, Bangor, for reading and criticising parts of the manuscript. Dr. Lou Hardy, Mr. John Fazey and Mr. Brian Rudall, of the University College of North Wales, Bangor, for supplying many valuable references. Miss Carolynn Rankin of the UK National Coaching Foundation for supplying up-to-date information on current research projects on the use of computers in sport. Dr. V. Parmar of the Royal Earlswood Hospital, Surrey, for supplying detailed information on the use of microcomputers by the Hospital to aid the handicapped. Dr. Jannneke Roos-Klein Lankhorst of the Agricultural University Hoallandse, Netherland, for supplying information on the use of computers in Landscape Design.

Special thanks to Mr. Terry Williams of the University College of North Wales, Bangor, for reading and supplying detailed criticism of the whole manuscript and for many valuable discussions throughout the writing.

Finally, I am very grateful indeed to Professor Myron Evans for his encouragement and for his very kind foreword.

Apart from the individuals mentioned above, many international companies and research institutions have also been very helpful in supplying information for the book. In particular, I would like to thank the following:

IBM UK, Wang Computers, BDH Ltd, Schnell Limited, Automatisme et Avenir Informatique, Nissen International, Soma Tech, Coto Research Centre and the Department of Medical Biophysics, University of Manchester.

Computers will play a critical role in delivering life-extension therapies. They will provide the "brain power" to regulate the flow of life-extending agents according to the needs of the body. Drugs and nutrients will be administered by small, computerised therapeutic systems - either implanted or applied externally - which will act like artificial organs to restore and maintain youthful homeostatic patterns within the body.

Saul Kent
In The Life-Extension Revolution.

Foreword

I was delighted to read this unique and wide-ranging book on a topic that is nearest to all our hearts. The book, through choosing to discuss health and fitness, sets out to show the human face of computers to the general reader and in my opinion, succeeds splendidly. It presents so much scientific information, yet it is all done in admirably lucid and easily readable style. It should be easily comprehensible to interested laypersons, as well as to specialists such as physicians, trainers in sporting activities and others who would like to have a broad perspective over the most vital applications of computers to their field.

Speaking as someone who has been involved in many aspects of computers and particularly of supercomputers, I was deeply impressed by the way Chapter 2 distilled accurately what a computer is and what is currently happening in the computer world. By pointing at the landmarks in the development of computing the chapter builds a historical perspective which is essential for understanding some of the reasons behind today's concerns and for speculating intelligently as to where the computer is going in the near future. In several instances, I noted how by laying bare the heart of the matter, the book manages to destroy the mystique of what is generally thought to be a highly technical subject. This, for example, is true of the description of Remote Sensing given in chapter 3.

In the last chapter, the suggestion that microcomputers should be used to extend the concept of exercise beyond mere muscular activity is eminently sensible. At present, the exercise programme of the average layperson caters for a very limited set of physiological and pscyhological functions and does not make use of personal data connected with the individual. Conventional procedures are geared to the needs of competitive sport and fashion, which of course are not the same as the needs of general health and preservation. The ideas developed in Chapter 4 try to remedy these failings and should prove particularly valuable in middle age and beyond when the brain becomes subject to deterioration if not used over the full range of its functions.

I have known Jan Abas for four years and over this period we have collaborated in research. I know that he has been highly active in using computers creatively in science, art, teaching and other fields. I know, for example, that he has used computers to model thermonuclear fusion as well as do Arabic calligraphy. He has used them to stimulate and encourage elderly persons and persons who are handicapped. As such he is highly qualified to tell the reader about a wide range of usages of computers. He is also highly qualified to propose novel uses as he has done in the last chapter of the book. I hope that many people will buy and read this book and that the book will encourage administrators and decision makers to give more thought to the use of technology for the improvement of the quality of human life.

M. W. Evans
IBM Corporation
Kingston, N.Y. 12401
July 1987.

Professor Myron Evans D.Sc. is a distinguished and multi-talented scientist. He has made many contributions to computer modelling of fundamental molecular processes and is the winner of the Harrison Memorial Prize and Meldola Medal of the Royal Society of Chemistry. He has authored more than 250 research papers and half a dozen state-of-the-art books. He is also a poet and an athlete. Professor Evans is currently a visiting professor at the world renowned IBM Research Centre at Kingston, New York.

1. Introduction

The computer is an incredibly versatile tool. The computer is not a pilot yet it can fly an aeroplane. It is not a telescope yet it can generate images of galaxies that are millions of light years away. It is not a detective yet it can outsniff any modern day Sherlock Holmes. For these reasons the computer has been called a generalised or a meta-medium, the first one invented by humans.

A major area of computer application that concerns everyone is that of health and fitness. Medicine, environmental sciences and sport are examples of topics in this area that are undergoing revolutionary changes through exploiting the power of the computer. This usage is bringing benefits to ordinary individuals as well as to those with special needs, such as champion athletes, astronauts and the most severely handicapped who can perhaps only wiggle a toe. Thanks to the computer we are learning to manage the life-support systems of our environment more wisely and are seeing the breathtakingly beautiful planet Earth in ways that it has never been seen before.

The computer is set to surpass today's methods of fighting disease in the way that the advances of 20th century medicine surpassed the wholesale application of bleeding and purging. Ultimately, through the developments now taking place in micro-electronics and micro-biology, the computer is destined to become the spearhead of evolution, consumating a new marriage of humans with machines. It constitutes the tool through which humans will radically extend their control over ageing and death.

Despite its extraordinary powers, versatility and promise the principles on which the computer operates are absurdly simple and can be grasped by anyone. These principles are very often obscured by technicalities and jargon. Although so much is written about the computer, many misconceptions continue to flourish. For example, despite its wondrous powers the computer is at present far from being a 'brain'. It would be generous to award the computer an IQ of, say, 5. The computer, despite its intimate association with micro-electronics is not inherently an electronics device. In the not-too-distant future computers will most probably be based on optics and work with beams of light.

The book first sets out to explain in a jargon-free language the nature of the computer and presents a complete overview of the key developments that are now taking place in the computer world. In the chapter that follows a wide-ranging non-technical survey shows how the computer is active in developing medicine, environmental sciences and sport.

In the final chapter we discuss how the computer might be exploited by the individual to construct a more sophisticated personalised programme of health and self preservation. The answer to the question - "Why use the computer in a general health programme?" can be given very succinctly. To preserve ourselves in the best possible shape we need to exercise all of the brain - not only the motor brain, which is the focus of concern in today's gymnasia, but also the sensory brain, the emotional brain, the intellectual brain and the memory-storing brain.

The computer can interact with the full spectrum of sensory information and can be readily adapted to cater for individual abilities, peculiarities and tastes. It can easily generate, collect, store and display useful information. It can cater for variety, novelty and surprise. Two hundred years ago Jean-Jacques Rousseau wrote, "Teach him to live rather than to avoid death: life is not breath but action, the use of our senses, mind, faculties, every part of ourselves which makes us conscious of our being". The last chapter discusses how, through the exploitation of the computer, it becomes possible at last to satisfy Rousseau's imperative and lift the gymnasium out of the "Pumping Iron" age, where it still resides.

Before we move on to singing the praise of the computer, it would be just as well, right at the start, to admit openly to the negative side of the coin. Computers are of course not without problems. In the wrong hands they can be a futile blind alley. Their employment is often expensive, particularly in staff costs. They bring fundamental problems of confidentiality and security. Much that is claimed by an average computer salesman can be pure hype. The author has worked continuously with computers of all shapes and sizes on a variety of applications for the last twenty years. He knows all the limitations and frustrations and is not so naive as to set out to suggest that computers are a panacea for all human ills. But then, there is no panacea for all human ills.

No one can deny that increasing reliance on computers over the full spectrum of human endeavour is quite inevitable. Whilst collecting material for this book the author was told a countless number of times, "I don't know how we managed without them". It would seem the wisest thing to do therefore to embrace the computer, to understand it and learn to rejoice in it.

It is easy, for persons bereft of any shreds of historical perspective, to adopt a stance against the 'evils' of technology. But the fact that those in the world who are without technology are desperate to acquire it is evidence enough that technology casts far more light than shadows. Deeper reflection shows that it is not technology but human wisdom and institutions which fail, leading to widespread disillusionment. It is humans who decide what technologies are developed and what use is made of them. The blame lies squarely with them and not with technology.

Whereas on the one hand humans display infinite eagerness to milk the cow of technology, on the other hand, as they do so they are inclined to whisper contemptuously in her ear, 'Go away, you are plundering our soul'. In keeping with this proclivity, the computer is perceived by many as a soulless device and no doubt under some circumstances the description is apt. But the computer is also making it possible to practice warmth, compassion and consideration in ways that are totally beyond the powers of a computer-less society. This, we hope, will be amply demonstrated in the book.

The book will be of value to all who wish to inform themselves of the role of the computer in the health of society. It will be of interest to members of the medical profession, the teaching profession, social and welfare organisers, to groups involved in various ways in health and sporting activities and to all those who care to see technology employed in the service of humankind for improving the quality of life. No familiarity with computers will be necessary to understand the material and all jargon and technical terms will be explained .

2. Key Concepts in Computer Appreciation

"Today we talked to our user group, booked our holiday, zapped nine monsters, checked the football results, bought two games, looked at share prices, learnt some French and conquered the Universe". So began an eye-catching advertisement in a computer magazine drumming out the fact that computers have now penetrated into every form of human endeavour. What is more, the developments so far may be likened to the tip of an iceberg. The tip is continuing to emerge at an ever increasing rate, revealing more and more of the iceberg and bringing with it extraordinary prospects for the future.

How is it that the computer has become so all pervasive in our lives with such astounding speed? Why is it that the computer is so infinitely adaptable? What makes it possible to fly spaceships, design artificial kidneys, model defence strategies and predict the world food shortage   all using the same tool ?

If we wish to understand the revolutionary changes now taking place in our world then it is essential to familiarise ourselves with the nature of the computer. Fortunately, the computer, despite its infinite versatility, or perhaps because of it, operates on principles that are easier to understand than the principles of operation of the four stroke engine that drives a car. Despite the Niagara of jargon that flows in computer sales literature, one need know nothing about electronics, 'ram', 'rom', 'computer languages', 'operating systems' etc. to appreciate the key principles that give the computer its power. Indeed, these principles, as we shall describe later, were discussed in depth by the British mathematician Alan Turing in 1937, long before the advent of modern electronics and long before the jargon was coined.

In this chapter our first object is to explain the fundamental nature of the computer to the general reader. We shall describe what a computer is and what a computer is not. We shall relate where the computer has come from and what is happening to it currently. The reader should be able to grasp fully the reasons for the versatilty of the computer. He should also be able to appreciate the reasons behind most major current research and development activity and recognise where the computer is going in the near future.

We hope that this understanding will help the reader who has previously been shy to feel enthusiastic about using this powerful tool in a creative way. In particular we hope that the reader will exploit the computer for personal development and growth and for the purposes of creating an autonomous programme of health and self preservation which is the subject of the last chapter in this book.

The Origins of Computer Power

Processing of codes

Imagine that you live on the top of a hill and would like to pass messages to someone who lives on another hill. Suppose that there is a single light on your door that is clearly visible to the other person, and suppose that you decide that the message to be passed will depend entirely on the state of the light being ON or OFF. Then clearly, this arrangement allows you to pass two distinct messages. For example, LIGHT ON could mean : 'there is a letter for you' and OFF that 'there is no letter for you '. Or that, 'the dog is still here' - 'the dog has run away'; 'meet me in the usual place' - ' can't make it tonight ' ; 'I want to see Jack' - 'I want to see Jill', etc.

The fundamental principle to grasp is that if a medium has two distinct states of functioning then we can associate two arbitrary distinct pieces of information with its functioning .

Exactly as the light bulb, the electronic computer operates with electrical components (mostly switches called transistors) that can be switched into adopting two different states. It is convenient to denote these states symbolically by the numbers 0 and 1 as we have done Fig. 2.1. What entity, operation or other kind of information is to be associated with the '0' and '1' is entirely dependent on the use we intend .

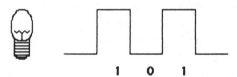

1   0   1

Fig 2.1.

Supposing now that we employ a set of two lights, rather than a single one, for transmitting our coded messages. It is easy to see that we can now transmit 2X2 or four distinct messages. Writing 'O' for OFF and * for ON, these are : OO, **, O* and *O. Similarly with a set of three lights we can make up 2X2X2 or eight messages, with eight lights 2X2X2X2X2X2X2X2 or 256 messages and so on.

We can see that by grouping a suitable number of two state components into convenient units we can make up codes to represent any number of operations, or any number of entities, or any number of operations involving any number of entities .

13

This is exactly how a computer operates. It is made up from two basic kinds of devices - logic elements (also called switching elements) and memory elements. The logic elements have two alternate pathways for currents to flow and memory elements have two different electrical states. These are grouped together in convenient numbers for operation. The smallest unit corresponding to the single light bulb in our analogy is called a BIT(Binary digIT). Eight bits grouped together are referred to as a BYTE. All operations and entities are coded in terms of 0's and 1's by utilising a suitable number of bytes.

A single byte can hold 256 different codes for anything we care to choose. For example, the so called ASCII code (American Standard Code for Information Interchange) - which is a commonly used code for encoding characters, assigns one byte for each character. This allows for the encoding of 256 different characters (although only 128 have been agreed so far). The letter 'A' is represented by the code 01000001, the semicolon ';' is represented as 00111010, etc.

It is important to appreciate that the same code could represent arbitrary 'things' or 'operations'. For example, the same pattern of 0's and 1's which is interpreted as the letter A in the context of characters is interpreted as the number 65 when dealing with integral numbers. In a different context it could be given some other meaning.

To make up an ad hoc example - we could associate each bit in a particular byte with the windows being CLEAN (=0) or DIRTY (=1) in an eight roomed house. In that case the ASCII code for the letter A (01000001) could be used to transmit the message 'Clean the windows in room numbers 7 and 1' to a robot window cleaner.

The fundamental reason for the versatility of the computer should now be clear. The computer is a device for the processing of coded information, whether the information relates to the evolution of galaxies or the functioning of a tin opener is quite immaterial.

It is also important to appreciate that the processing of coded information is ultimately the most fundamental mode of functioning. Life itself, at the profoundest level, functions via coded information. The DNA molecule - a long complex chain forming the genes in the cells of all living creatures - is a code for transmitting information from one generation to the next. Our brain is a code processing device that transforms the codes generated by the nervous impulses from the external world into information about our reality.

An example

Let us now look at a real example to illustrate how the code processing action is utilised in a practical application. We shall use this example to crystallise all the key features of the computer.

One major application of computers is in generating pictures. Computer pictures are used by scientists, artists, businessmen and school children, to name but a few. Let us see how the coding process is turned into the creation of pictures .

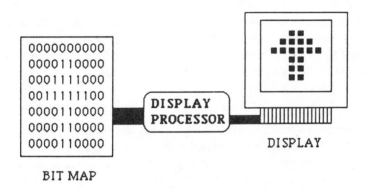

BIT MAP

Fig 2.2.

Fig 2.2 shows how a monochrome (single colour) picture is displayed on a TV-like display by a modern computer graphics work station. The display screen is divided into dots called PIXELS (meaning picture elements). Each pixel comprises a tiny coating of material that emits light when struck with a beam of electrons, which happens when the pixel ON (=1) code is sent by the computer to a device known as the display processor. The code for the image is stored in an area of the computer's memory called the bit map.

In a monochrome display a pixel can only be ON or OFF. All we need do to code the image is to allocate one bit to each pixel. If the bit is 1 then the pixel is ON, and if it is zero then the pixel is OFF. To generate the picture we simply send lines of 0's and 1's to the display processor. Whenever a '1' is received a burst of electrons is emitted and the appropriate pixel is lit up. The total number of lit up pixels at any time make up the complete picture. This process is repeated over and over again to keep the image updated on the screen. Fig. 2.2 shows an arrow being displayed.

At this stage it should be easy to work out what is required if we want to display a multi-intensity or a multi-colour image. We now need to associate more bits with each pixel : 2 bits per pixel will allow the coding of 4 different intensities or colours; 1 byte or 8 bits per pixel will allow 256 possibilities for intensity levels and colours, etc. This is exactly what is done to produce colour or shaded images.

Typically, a simple colour graphics system allocates three bits to each pixel and the state of each bit is used to drive 3 beams that generate the three primary colours Red, Green and Blue. Thus if the bits corresponding to red and green are ON then

15

this results in yellow. The 3-bit coding scheme allows the naming of 8 colours, which are usually chosen as black, green, blue, cyan, red, magenta, yellow and white. More versatile systems utilise more bits to code the colour variation of each pixel. For example 8 bits per pixel, giving 256 colours, is quite common in professional work.

Clearly, to generate our picture, we need some means of getting the code for the picture into the computer. We need to store the code somewhere and we need to be able to process the code so as to change the picture in some way - to move it, to rotate it, to magnify or shrink it etc. These requirements define the nature of the other components of the computer.

Memory

The very simple picture displayed in Fig. 2.2 has 70 pixels. Its code is stored in 10 rows of bits with 7 bits per row. Thus to be able to generate this picture the computer needs 70 bits of internal 'memory' for 'data'. The memory requirements for the data in this example are very small but the purpose of this component should be clear.

A more realistic display, if it is to appear anything like smooth, would require many more pixels and demand many more bits. The human eye needs about 90 dots per inch in a figure to overcome the sense of jaggedness and see it as being smooth.

Typically, a cheap home computer in 1987 might offer a resolution of 300 X 300 pixels and a good professional display would offer something nearer to 1000 X 1000. Thus a professional display that allocated 8 bits per pixel, would need 8 X 1000 X 1000 or 8 million bits (8M bits) to store the image (the DATA) of our picture. Clearly we would also need storage for the instructions (the PROGRAM) to process the picture and room for codes that supervise the general functioning (the SYSTEMS SOFTWARE) of the computer.

We can now appreciate one of the major practical requirements of a general purpose computer that deals in long and unwieldy strings of 0's and 1's. It needs a large memory. A technological component that has brought power to the modern computer arises from its facility to store vast amounts of information compactly in its primary internal memory and from being able to access very much more via other compact secondary storage devices such as magnetic tapes and disks.

Speed Requirements

Returning to our graphics example, it is easy to appreciate that to change a picture in a real display we need to calculate the bit pattern of several million bits. Also, to draw the picture on the display we need to be able to transmit information about the same millions of bits to the display processor. Clearly, if these tasks are to be accomplished in seconds then we need great speeds of computation and transmission.

The facility to process coded information is by itself only a theoretical source of power. It is only when codes kept in large memories are accessed, executed and transmitted accurately and at great speeds that the computer begins to possess the essential components that combine to make it something special. Computers are powerful because even the humblest of them is able to perform millions of operations with absolute accuracy in a second. This is possible because the logic and the memory elements of the computer can change their state in times of the order of a millionth or even a billionth of a second.

We can now appreciate that although using light bulbs, we could in theory achieve by hand anything that an electronic computer can do, it would take us millions of times longer. If a hand operated switch were used to change the state of a device every second then it would take about twelve days of non-stop pressing to achieve what the humblest machine can do in a second. Also, if a human were to make only one mistake per million additions, say, then such a human would be regarded as infallible and possessed of miraculous powers. If a computer were to achieve the same rate of 'success' then it would have to be pronounced an utter failure since it would be producing a mistake every second.

Input - Output (The user interface)

Returning once again to our example, we will now introduce some further essential components. These, from the point of view of the user, happen to be the most important ones.

Clearly we need to be able to tell the computer in some way what picture we want it to draw. We may also wish to interact with the picture when it is on display. We may, for example, wish to rotate it, zoom into a selected portion, change the colour of a piece, etc. We need to be able to INPUT information from the user into the machine.

We also need the machine to OUTPUT the picture on various devices. We may want it on a TV monitor, a piece of paper or we may wish to store it on a floppy disc for future viewing.

A computer is only useful if it can communicate effectively with the outside world. It needs to be able to receive information (INPUT) and give information back after processing (OUTPUT).

In the beginning the INPUT/OUTPUT operations were carried out entirely by means of punched paper tape or cards in the language of 0's and 1's understood by the computer. This was painfully cumbersome and may have been the reason for a howler committed by Professor Aitken, an early British pioneer of computing, who speculated that "perhaps we shall need 3 computers and a few highly trained mathematicians to satisfy the entire computing requirements of U.K. "

It is easy to appreciate that the extent to which computers can be effectively utilised by large numbers of people is entirely dependent on the ease of HUMAN/MACHINE communication. The reason why millions of home micros have been sold is that any child can learn how to load a game and enjoy zapping aliens by merely pressing a few buttons or twiddling some knobs. Equally, the reason why millions of home micros remain under utilised and gather dust is that the user interface for tasks other than zapping aliens is not as yet in a very convenient form.

It is equally important to appreciate that what we attach to the computer on the input and output side is dependent entirely on our ingenuity in designing appropriate devices for turning some actions into codes and some codes into actions . We give below an example of an unconventional mode of input to clarify the meaning of this remark.

Dr. Peter Griffiths of St George's Hospital, Lincoln, U.K. and his associates have developed an ingenious interface for the use of some very severely disabled people. It uses only the eye movement for input. The eye muscles carry a small electrical charge and as they move a tiny electric current is generated. This current is detected by electrodes worn on the user's head. The current is then turned into a code to move a cursor on a computer menu. This interface has made communication possible for some who were previously almost entirely cut off from the world and was awarded a prize by the British Computer Society.

Yet another source of computer power arises from the fact that there is no restriction on the kind of input and output devices that can be attached to it. It is for this reason that the computer can be made to fire a missile, bake a cake, type a letter or play a symphony.

Algorithms

No portrait of the computer would be complete if it failed to highlight the significance of SOFTWARE. A computer is to computing what a musical instrument is to music. Just as no violin can give an indication of the melodies that may be played on it, so the finest computer can accomplish absolutely nothing without the software. It is the software that ultimately puts the computer's orchestra of components to play the desired tune in harmony.

The software comprises a collection of algorithms. These are a series of instructions or procedural steps designed to achieve the solution of a problem. Some of the algorithms are for general purpose tasks required of a machine, such as receiving information from a keyboard or filing information on disks. These are written by specialists and are called SYSTEMS SOFTWARE. Another class of algorithms are those that are meant for some special application such as word processing. These are again written by professionals and are called APPLICATIONS PACKAGES. Finally there are algorithms written by individual users to achieve their special ends. These are individual PROGRAMS.

All algorithms are made up from the following kinds of commands:

Begin
    Do task A
    Do task B
    ....
    If X is true then do task C otherwise do task D
    Repeat task E until Y becomes false
    If Z is true then go back to step N and start again
    If W is true then jump forward to step M
    ....
End

These commands are executed by the PROCESSOR. The execution comprises arithmetical and logical operations on the strings of 0's and 1's kept in the internal memory and the operations of input and output with the external environment.

Thus, to employ a computer to ring an alarm bell when the temperature goes above 80 degrees in a room, we might proceed as follows. Firstly, we need a device that can turn the temperature measured by some means in the room, such as a thermometer, into numerical information. Such a device is called an ADC (analog to digital converter). This information would be input to the computer at regular intervals and deposited as a string of 0's and 1's in some internal memory location. The algorithm would involve fetching this information from the memory location, examining to see if the value exceeds 80 (a logical operation), and sending an appropriate code to a DAC (digital to analog converter - which in this case would be an alarm bell) if it became true.

We see that the computer does not do anything at all that is very complicated. Just as through the simple but repeated action of combining the 26 letters of the alphabet in groups to form words we can produce the works of Shakespeare, so it is that the computer by merely doing inputs, outputs and simple arithmetical and logical operations on strings of 0's and 1's can accomplish what appears miraculous. The complexity is always handled by the computer by breaking it down into a multitude of simple steps. This is the case when it is used for such complicated tasks as designing a Jumbo Jet or forecasting the weather.

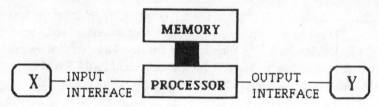

Fig 2.3.

A Model for the Computer

We have now described all the key components of a computer. These are pictured abowe in Fig. 2.3. A summary of the discussion follows.

Summary

A computer has a processor for processing codes which reside in its memory. We can attach anything X to a computer e.g. a human, a thermometer, a tape recorder or a monkey, so long as we can devise an interface for turning some consistent action by X into codes involving strings of 0's and 1's and so long as we can devise a set of rules for interpreting and processing these codes. Similarly we can attach anything Y e.g., a TV, a printer, a burglar alarm, a mouse cage etc. on the output side so long as we can devise an interface for turning the 0's and 1's given out by the computer to activate Y in a consistent way.

The power of the computer comes from universal qualities underlying its hardware and software. Both the hardware and software handle complexities by breaking them down into simple operations that can be executed repeatedly at great speeds.

Although our model in Fig. 2.3 shows only single units, in practice there may be several processors, memory units and input and output devices.

Where has the Computer come from?

We have now seen what a computer is. We now want to broaden our appreciation and as with any subject, this is best achieved in the context of a historical perspective. In this section we shall trace the evolution of the computer and see where it has come from.

Since the processing of coded information is the most fundamental activity of life processes, one would expect that the invention of devices that function in this way would have a long history. That indeed is the case. The drums and smoke signals of primitive man, the development of writing, the use of morse and semaphore signalling are just a few examples of such inventions. However, in these examples the 'processing' aspect is only rudimentary. The actions of combining coded information to obtain new information or information in a very different format make greater demands on processing.

When it comes to devices for processing of codes, the inventions of the past have been aimed mostly at numerical information. The computing devices of the past have been calculators. The reason for this lies in the practical needs of the past and in the fact that the rules for combining of numerical codes are defined in a very exact and obvious way (2+2 = 4). Thus to trace the evolution of the present day computer we have, for the most part, to trace the history of calculators. This we shall now do very briefly. In what follows, we shall see how at each stage the current technology has placed limits on the power and universality of the code processing devices of the day.

The earliest calculating device invented by humans made use of the ready-made fingers and toes. Soon pebbles, cowrie shells and similar small discrete objects were introduced. The first purpose-built calculator was the abacus, invented in China around 2500 B.C. and still very much in use by some sections of the population in the Far East. No other calculating device of any significance was invented for the next 4000 years.

For the next noteworthy inventions we must turn to 17th century Europe. In 1617 the Scotsman John Napier devised his 'Napier's bones' which employed logarithmic scales to perform multiplications and divisions. This offered a very useful labour saving device and was the progenitor of the slide rule which was the widespread tool used for scientific calculations until cheap electronic pocket calculators became available.

On the continent of Europe, around 1640, Blaise Pascal, the French mathematical prodigy employed toothed gear wheels in the design of the first mechanically driven calculator. This was a significant advance and Pascal, appropriately, is honoured by having one of the major modern computer languages named after him. The technology of 17th century Europe was, however, not as yet sufficiently advanced to be able to produce gear wheels and other such components of high precision. Pascal's computer, though improved by the Swiss mathematician Leibniz, remained for a long time a mere curiosity.

Then in the 1820s the Englishman Charles Babbage began working on plans to produce mechanical calculators. He designed a 'Difference Engine' for the automatic production of mathematical tables but soon moved on to dream of bigger and better things. In the mid-19th century he proposed an automatic 'Analytical Engine'. This was intended to be a general purpose device capable of performing by mechanical means any sequence of arithmetical calculations which a mathematician could do. Babbage devoted the rest of his life to his Engine and to the improvement of technology of gears that would drive it.

Although Babbage failed to complete his Engine, he went a long way in elucidating the fundamental processes involved in the activity of calculation. In particular, he realised the importance of the repeat and the conditional instruction - 'REPEAT so and so UNTIL so and so', 'IF so and so THEN so and so ELSE so and so' which are part and parcel of every modern computer language. Lady Ada Lovelace, daughter of the poet Lord Byron, and Babbage's devoted disciple, was also the first to propose a program to be stored in the calculator and be capable of modification at will. She too has a modern programming language named after her.

As technology improved, the early 20th century saw the development of several more robust mechanical and electro-mechanical calculators. In the late 1930s Professor Howard H. Aiken of Harvard university developed the first automatic calculator which he called the 'Automatic Sequence Controlled Calculator' and which later became known as 'Mark I'. The machine could receive instructions via punched cards, punched tapes or a series of switches. The calculator worked using electro-mechanical relays for switching and took about a 1/3rd of a second to perform an addition.

The same era also produced some highly significant theoretical work on machine calculation. Outstanding amongst these was the work of Turing. Turing invented the concept of the abstract computing machine, now known as the Turing machine. The machine consists of an imaginary paper tape divided into squares along its length. The squares can be inscribed with codes. It works by passing one square at a time to the left or right across a head where the operations of reading, writing and erasing the codes can be carried out. With this simple arrangement Turing brilliantly isolated the notions of internal processing, a stored program executed sequentially, storage and retrieval through a read/write head and input and output. In doing so the Turing machine abstracted all the fundamental features of computers as they exist today. It distilled all the rules which must be obeyed in the workings of any computational machine. For these reasons, the machine remains a powerful model for thinking deeply about computation and provides a standard vehicle for logical thought in computer science.

It was not until technology became available to allow for the generation, transmission, amplification and switching of electrical signals at a very much faster rate than could be achieved mechanically or electro-mechanically that the modern electronic computer could be born. It was the invention of the vacuum tube, which made possible the control of electricity by electronic rather than electro-mechanical means, that provided the key component. Although the vacuum tube had been invented in 1906 it was the Second World War that provided the impetus to develop the kind of complex circuitry that could be utilised in an electronic computer.

The most powerful of the early electronic computers named Colossus was produced in 1943 by a British team which included Turing. The computer was designed to break the so called 'Enigma codes' which were codes employed by the German armed forces for transmission of military information. Colossus contained about 15000 valves (vacuum tubes) and could process 25000 characters per second. The reader should note that this machine was designed to process non-numerical information and not for performing arithmetical operations (it is generally proclaimed that the first electronic computers were designed to do arithmetical calculations).

Another special purpose machine known as ENIAC (Electronic Numerical Integrator and Calculator) was constructed by electrical engineers Presper Eckert and John Mauchly at the University of Pennsylvania between 1942 and 1945 for computing artillery range tables. It contained something like 18000 valves and could do an addition in about 1/5000 of a second. ENIAC was wired to perform a set sequence of calculations and required extensive rewiring to perform a fresh set of calculations.

The work on ENIAC led to something very fortunate for computing. In 1944 John von Neumann, one of the leading mathematicians of this century, who was at the time involved with calculations on the Atom Bomb visited Eckert and Mauchly. He became fired with the desire to improve ENIAC. Von Neumann set out to produce the logical design of an electronic computer that could store its program, a program that could be changed instantly without requiring any rewiring of the machine. During 1945-46 von Neumann and his collaborators published a series of reports which crystallised the architecture of a general purpose electronic computer as we know it today. Von Neumann's initial ideas, particularly in the form of sequential processing, have stamped their mark on the manner in which computers have developed over the decades. His thinking has permeated not only the hardware of the machine but also the way programming has evolved. As we shall see later, the next generation of computers may at last be able to shed von Neumann's legacy but today's computer, despite revolutionary advances in electronics, continues to be referred to by computer specialists as 'the von Neumann machine'.

The first stored program computers were produced round about 1947 in several laboratories in Britain and USA. The Eckert-Mauchly UNIVAC, which reached the market in 1950, was the first commercial computer.

Vacuum tubes, or valves, had crucial limitations. They were bulky, consumed large amounts of power and produced large amounts of heat. Any large configurations placed severe limits on reliability. Before reliable circuits of much greater complexity could be built, a jump forward in technology had to take place. This came with the invention of the transistor at the Bell Telephone Laboratory in 1947. The transistor offered not only a much smaller and faster switch for generating the ON-OFF or the 0s and 1s for the machine but it consumed a million times less power.

In the late 1950s Integrated Circuits, circuits in which transistors and other electrical components are fabricated all together on a semiconductor chip, were developed. Silicon supplied the cheapest of the chip materials. The combination of smallness, fastness and cheapness opened the flood gates of information processing. Thus what began with fingers, toes and pebbles proceded via mechanical, electro-mechanical, and electronic means and is presently at the stage of being driven by microelectronics. No doubt the progression will continue and the driving medium will take other forms.

The Current Scene

The extraordinarily rapid development of the computer over the last 25 or 30 years is unprecedented. It is said that had the aircraft industry undergone a similarly spectacular evolution during the same period then a Jumbo Jet would cost only about £200 today, would circle the globe in less than 15 minutes and consume less than 5 gallons of fuel. This pace of change makes it very difficult to retain a perspective of the proliferating technological wizardry.

Despite that, it is our intention in this section to offer the general reader a broad perspective over the key developments that are taking place currently. We shall describe the scene in terms of four different themes:

1. Computers and related devices are becoming smaller, lighter, cheaper and faster in operation.

2. The densities and the capacities of memory units, both internal and external, are growing.

3. Communication between computers and humans and between computers and other devices, including other computers, is becoming faster and more extensive.

4. Through the marriage of the above three processes it is becoming possible to evolve and employ a more extensive range of algorithms to tackle a more extensive range of tasks. Of particular significance is the emergence of knowledge-based systems.

The above processes are of course all highly interdependent for their evolution. However, by categorising them in this way it becomes possible to reduce the complexity of the electronic jungle and bring the picture into some sort of managable focus.

Smaller-lighter-cheaper-faster

In the last 30 years or so computational speeds have increased on average by a factor of 2000 and what would have taken a year to do on computers of the fifties can now be done on the fastest computers in seconds. In the same period the price has decreased by a factor of 1,000 and equipment that can now be carried in a small briefcase would have occupied a huge room to be able to perform similarly. This trend continues.

The speed at which computers operate depends on a number of factors. It depends on the rate at which individual components can switch their state. It depends on the rate at which various interlinked units can communicate and it depends on the way the information is organised and shared. Overall progress is being made through advances on all these fronts.

The top ratings for speeds of computation have until very recently been held by the so called SUPERCOMPUTERS. These machines are used for weather forecasting, aircraft design and other complex and mathematically demanding tasks. Until very recently the term supercomputer has been synonymous with two machines named Cyber and Cray. Both of these have been designed by American companies, the first by Control Data Corporation (CDC) and the second by Cray Research. The first versions of these supercomputers appeared in mid 70's.

More recently Japanese companies Fujitsu, NEC and Hitachi have all produced their own versions of high performance supercomputers to challenge the American monopoly.

There are two common yardsticks for measuring computer speeds. The MIPS rating (millions of instructions per second) measures the rate at which the processor executes instructions. The other is the FLOPS rating (floating point operations per second) which measures the number of arithmetical sums the computer can perform per second.

CRAY 1 which appeared in the mid 70's is rated at 150 Megaflops (150 million sums per second). CRAY 2 which appeared in 1985 is 12 times faster and 50% lighter and by linking four of them it is possible to do up to 7200 million arithmetical calculations per second.

Cray 3 due in the early 1990's will use the faster switching material gallium arsenide instead of silicon and will be many times faster. The newest supercomputer designed by CDC, named ETA 10, has just appeared and is rated at 10 Gigaflops or 10,000 million arithmetical sums per second and so the race goes on.

Supercomputers achieve their high performance in three main ways. Firstly, they employ very fast components. Secondly, they are very compactly designed to reduce the travel time for electrical signals to move from one point to another. The Cray X-MP/48 which is currently the most powerful of the Crays occupies only six square metres of floor space. Thirdly, supercomputers contain special hardware designed to process vectors (strings of numbers) in contrast with conventional computers which handle individual numbers. Some of these machines also exploit the 'parallel mode' of operation whereby independent tasks are performed simultaneously through a number of linked processors. The X-MP/48, for example, contains four processors in one box. These can be run as four independent machines or can be made to cooperate on a single job. Parallelism is a very important concept for the future and the reader should take special note of its meaning.

The techniques exploited by supercomputers are now emerging on medium size and small microcomputers. An exciting example of this trend is the Transputer, manufactured by the U.K. company Inmos. It was first announced in 1983 and marketed in October 1985. The Transputer's design places the processor unit and the memory unit on a single chip which measures less than 9mm square on which there are packed 200,000 transistors.

The Transputer is made using a technology called complementary metal oxide silicon (CMOS) which consumes less power, generates less heat and allows for faster switching of state than those achieved by the conventional silicon. It has a parallel (or concurrent) processor, which simply means that the processor can carry out several computations simultaneously.

The design of the Transputer not only gives high speeds of processing, but makes it possible for Transputers to be linked together in clusters to function in parallel. In this way it has been possible to attain speeds comparable with those of supercomputers, but at a vastly reduced price. A single transputer costs under £350 and a linked cluster costing under £10,000 has been able to do certain calculations at speeds of a Cray 2 which costs £13 million.

Other similar developments make it certain that computers powerful enough to design space vehicles and to model nuclear explosions will, in the not-too-distant future, become affordable by average persons and will sit on desk tops.

Higher density and higher capacity memory units

The same technologies that lead to faster speeds are at work to increase densities and capacities of memory units. Silicon memory chips that are used for internal memories have increased their capacity from 1k (1000 bits) to 64k in a period of ten years and 256k chips are now commonly on the market. At the time of writing this book the most advanced commercially available memory chip is the one-megabit DRAM. However, the Japnese company Nippon Telegraph has already announced a prototype 16-megabit chip which is capable of storing more information than goes into 600 pages of typewritten text. Judging by the present rate of progress, by early next century chips capable of storing up to 64 megabits will be commonplace.

External storage devices are similarly expanding in capacity. A vastly more capacious device compared to the magnetic disk is the Laser Optical Disk. The disk is written using a laser beam which burns tiny slots in plastic and produces densities up to ten times those attained on a magnetic disk.

An American company has transcribed an entire nine million word encyclopedia on such a disk and when connected to an IBM PC or similar micro the system has given average search times of less than five seconds for the entries.

A serious limitation of the present version of the optical disk is that it cannot be wiped to record new information repeatedly. However, new processes of recording are expected to overcome this problem and this kind of external storage medium is expected to become the one in common use.

Easier, more effective human/machine communication

The ultimate objective in information processing is for humans to make sense of information. Not surprisingly, research and development to improve effectiveness in communication occupies one of the most central positions in computing.

The first significant extension in human/machine communication occurred in the mid 1960s with the invention of time-sharing. This made it possible for many users to share a computer simultaneously. It was then that the first crude terminals called Teletypes, which clatteringly punched out 10 characters per second, got wired up to centrally sited computers. Soon the reels of punched tapes and boxes of punched cards that had been precious hall marks of computer people became worth less than their weight in salvage. The Teletypes brought the computer user the first taste of instant (well almost instant) response by the computer.

The interface has been transformed beyond recognition in only a few years. Today we have desk-top computers powerful enough to display and manipulate not only characters but also images. Laser printers, which can quietly and quickly produce crisp and clear images, are about to put an end to the last remnants of mechanical clattering. Many other kinds of devices and methods, such as mice, joysticks, networks, electronic mail etc., which make communication easier and more effective have rapidly evolved.

Improvements in communication result from three kinds of developments. Firstly, through the attachment of devices to the computer that take advantage of the more natural functioning of the human brain and body. Secondly, through the improvement of the manner of display of information on these devices and thirdly through the development of hardware and software that allows computers to communicate with other computers more speedily. Each of these makes it possible to handle complex information more easily and speedily.

Graphics

Perhaps as much as two thirds of the brain is involved in the processing of visual information. Not surprisingly, it is frequently exclaimed that a picture is worth a thousand words. Pictures drawn by cavemen depict vividly that humans have relied on images to represent concepts from earliest of times.

Undoubtedly, the most significant advance in human/machine communication has come through the use of computer graphics. Efforts to attach graphics devices to computers began almost as soon as the computer was invented, but until about 1976 computer graphics remained specialised and expensive. It conveyed for most people - no more than Snoopy printed in patterns of stars and crosses.

It was the Apple II costing £2000 in 1976 which initially made colour graphics available at a price that was affordable by many. The first interactive graphics terminal, the IBM 2250, marketed in 1965, had a price tag of more than £50,000, but today for under £100 it is possible to buy a micro that can do far more.

Despite its recent introduction, the impact of computer graphics has been all embracing. Scientists, artists, businessmen, designers, engineers, medics and school children are examples of users who have all been able to use computers more effectively in this way. For this reason, computer graphics is today a multi-million pound industry and one of the key growth areas in computing.

User-friendliness and user-centredness

Presenting information in pictorial form so that it can be absorbed quickly and effectively is only one example of 'user-friendliness'. There is much more to it. Truly effective human/machine communication demands a range of facilities that allow the user to interact as naturally as possible with the computer. The user should be able to tailor the computer easily for his specific needs and make it do his bidding. This is the goal of the human/machine interface designers.

Everyone can learn to handle the complexity of the car because the interface involves only such components as the steering wheel and the clutch pedal which demand simple natural responses. In the same way, many more persons could learn to handle the complexity of the computer if the interface were designed to demand only simple actions rather than the learning of special languages or the memorising of long and involved commands.

The difficulty, however, is that whereas the car is used only for the purposes of going from A to B, the computer is used for an unlimited number of tasks. The design of an effective computer interface is therefore a much tougher problem. However, major improvements have taken place in the last few years. The interface is being designed to respond to easier and more natural actions and more thought is being given to the characteristics of the user's environment.

The biggest jump in this direction, which set the trend for the future, occured in 1984 with the launch of the APPLE MACINTOSH microcomputer. It combined graphics with a hand operated device called the mouse and offered a menu-selectable command language. The Macintosh was the first machine to be packaged and marketed as an 'appliance' in much the same way as a car, a washing machine or a TV set is an appliance for whose usage no specialist knowledge is needed.

For many standard applications, such as wordprocessing, no specialist knowledge whatsoever is required to operate the Macintosh. When an applications program is run, a menu bar appears on top of the screen and displays the names of all the functions available to the user. The user selects a function from this menu bar by rolling a small hand held device called the mouse to point at the function and pressing a button on the mouse when the choice is reached. This causes a list of all possible actions associated with that command to appear on the screen below the pointer. Keeping the mouse button pressed, the user then moves the pointer over the desired action and releases the button. The computer obeys.

Some tasks require additional information from the user. In that case a 'dialog box' appears which is again manipulated using the mouse, with possibly some small amount of typing. The user is given ample opportunity to make corrections, or cancel or undo the effects of a command. General tasks, such as deleting files, are also easily performed through pointing at 'icons'. These are easily deciphered pictorial representations. Typically, to delete a file, one uses the mouse to drag the icon for the file into an area occupied by a dustbin shaped icon.

An example of concern for the needs of the individual user is shown by the Sensor Work Station, being developed by the Japanese company Mitsubishi. The Sensor's ergonomic design adds a personal touch to what the Macintosh offers in allowing the work station to be tailored to suit the height, weight, eyesight and other personal characteristics of the user.

Taking account of the user's environment has led to other concepts for the improvement of the interface. For example, it is a fact that in the working environment one is constantly interrupted. The telephone rings, someone knocks at the door, a manual has to be found, coffee time arrives and so on. To cater for the fact that a user cannot be expected to attend to a single task for long periods, equipment is being designed that allows for easy switching between a number of tasks.

An example of this is the launch in 1985 by the U.K. company ICL of its OPD (one per desk) computer. For about £1500 the OPD comes not only with the usual computer, the display, the keyboard and the disk drives, but also includes a telephone and a modem(for access to other computers) in a single integrated unit. The OPD can attend to up to eight different tasks simultaneously.

Machine/machine communication

Information should ideally be available when it is needed and where it is needed. Linking of computers into networks is therefore, understandably, another major growth area.

The simplest device for computer/computer communication is the modem (short for modulator/demodulator) which sends information across ordinary telephone lines. Modems can be used to dial up other computers with modems, or to link into larger communication networks.

Typically, modems are used by travelling businessmen to carry a portable office and keep in touch with the central site. Another growing use of modems is in the sending and receiving of electronic mail. In this method, the mail is sent to a central computer which then posts it into a mailbox. It then becomes available for reading by any authorised person who is in possession of the right password.

Modems in common use are slow devices. The typical rate at which they communicate is 300 baud (bits per second) although the state-of-the-art ones can achieve 9600 baud. Faster networks work at baud rates of several million.

Next to the appearance of the microcomputer, the most important technology to emerge is undoubtedly that of the Local Area Networks (LAN). LANs allow resources to be shared and a variety of dissimilar devices to communicate at high speeds. Typically, a secretary sitting in one office can print out a letter on a high quality printer in another office or access a file jointly with ten others.

The best-known LAN system at present is the American system Ethernet operating at 10 megabaud. Each Ethernet LAN can spread over 500 metres and can connect 100 devices. Five of these can be joined together to form a network covering 2.5 kilometres and connecting 1024 devices.

Artificial Intelligence

Despite their wonderous powers, today's computers have severe limitations. Although they are unmatchable by the human brain in storing, retrieving and performing billions of accurate calculations and inferences, they can only process precisely represented information using precisely defined algorithms. The computer cannot cope with imprecise information or lack of an algorithm in ways that are absolutely elementary for the human brain.

The brain, for example, has no difficulty in recognising Fig 2.4 (a) as human faces despite the crudity and distortions. In (b), the large number of variations to represent the same letter present no difficulty either. Only partial information is instantly recognised in (c) and (d). By seizing on the context, identical blobs in (e) and (f) are deciphered as fish in one case and birds in another. These are just a few examples of the way the human brain excells over the computer.

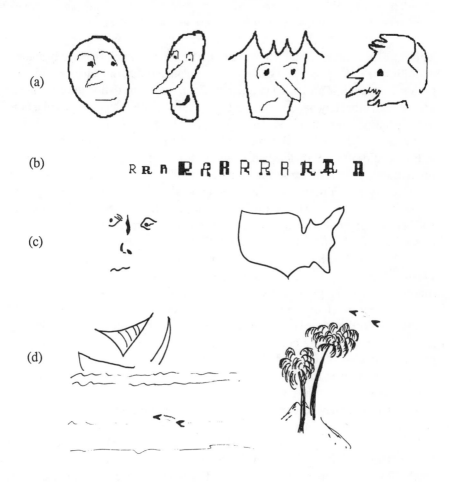

(a)

(b)

(c)

(d)

Fig 2.4.

A computer is not a brain. As we said earlier, it would be very generous to grant the mightiest computers of today an IQ of 5. Intelligence implies the ability to cope with imprecise information. It implies the ability to extract salient features from a mass of information. Intelligence gives power to organise and classify information. Intelligence is holistic and seizes quickly upon the meaning of a piece of information through summing up its context. These skills are as yet not possessed by computers to any significant degree.

Since the early 40's researchers have set out to try to endow machines with all the above attributes, albeit starting from very meagre beginnings. It is asserted that the computer need not remain capable only of solving problems that demand calculative rationality. A computer, the researchers proclaim, can have increasing amounts of what humans call common sense and intelligence.

The quest goes back to Turing, the pioneer theoretician of computer science whom we mentioned earlier. He was among the first to think rigorously about the definition of intelligence and came to the conclusion that machines could indeed perform in ways that are called intelligent. Even before the deliberations of Turing, a number of other key papers appeared in the early 1940s which proposed methods to build 'purposeful' machines. These papers showed how machines could perform abstractions and could employ models and analogies to solve problems.

By the mid-50's, computers had acquired sufficient speed and storage capacities for researchers to start exploring some of the ideas of machine intelligence in a rudimentary way. Programs were written that allowed computers to play a good game of checkers, prove theorems in geometry and do other things which until then had been considered to be in the exclusive domain of human intelligence. This taste of success gave birth to the subject of Artificial Intelligence (AI).

The history of AI has been a highly controversial one. Much spurious debate of the form 'can a machine really be intelligent ?' - 'well it all depends what you mean by intelligence ', 'can pigs really fly ? - 'well it all depends on how you define pigs and how you measure flying ', etc., has been conducted between the enthusiasts and the detractors. Workers in AI have been accused of 'playing with toys' and 'indulging in a genuine stupidity', amongst other such hurled insults. Equally, some AI enthusiasts have proclaimed that the very existence of America, or Western Civilisation, or even the Human Race depends entirely on the amplitude of funds allocated to AI research. This debate goes on.

The facts lie somewhere in between. 'Playing with toys' is exactly how an entirely new notion can take root. Galileo played with pendulums and balls, Newton played with prisms; Faraday played with magnets and the Wright brothers played with a wire and fabric flying contraption. Their toys, nevertheless, matured to change the world. Since machine intelligence is a radically new concept, the pioneers would necessarily have to start with toys.

It is true though that the AI enthusiasts have often overblown their successes and their projections have usually been over optimistic. Undoubtedly, there is a long road ahead for AI yet and it is clear that the present day 'von Neumann' machine is not well suited to replicate the cognitive processes of the brain.

Brains differ in operation from the present day computer in striking ways. The nerve cells, or neurons, are individually a million times slower than the transistor but they are far more numerous and far more richly connected. The wiring patterns of neurons have complexities of a different order all together; one cell may receive input from as many as 100,000 others. The neurons do not process information serially like a von Neumann machine but whole collections work in parallel. These are just a few of the differences.

New jumps in technology as well as methods of organising and processing information are needed before AI can truly deliver such goods as speech and pattern recognition which defy compact algorithmic description. This is not to say that AI efforts directed on the present day machines have been wasted. As Dr. Fredrico Faggin, the man who designed the first microprocessor (the Intel 4004) put it recently, ' AI has made a tremendous contribution in making us understand how difficult the problem is. Just to understand that takes a lot of work.'

We shall return to AI in the next section when we come to describe the concept of the Fifth Generation computer. We refer the interested reader to references [4], [5], [8] and [9] which contain whole series of claims and counter claims in AI made by opposing champions. We shall now describe 'knowledge-based' systems which are at present the most mature products of AI that are in practical use.

Knowledge-based or expert systems

Knowledge-based systems, also called expert systems, are designed to deal with complexities in the way that has traditionally been done by human experts.

To understand what they do, let us first recognise two different kinds of complexities. There is the kind of complexity involved in flying an aeroplane. During flight there are many mechanical and electrical components to observe and respond to, but the individual behaviour of each component is well understood. This is organisational complexity and arises through rapid interaction of many components in a complex way. The human expert in such situations needs to possess quickness of responses and clear deterministic rules of procedure.

The other kind of complexity is the kind met in law or medicine. It comes with 'if...then perhaps... maybe...but then again it could mean so and so...on the other hand it might be the case.."... This complexity arises through lack of determinism in the situation and the inability to obtain complete knowledge. Here the human expert functions to increase the probability of achieving the desired ends .

Both kinds of complexities are widespread in real life situations and expert systems are increasingly being employed to handle both of them.

The first kind of complexity is easier to deal with and has been the domain of computers for a considerable time. This application has usually been called 'process control'. The operation of nuclear power stations, distribution of electricity, control of robots and machine tools in various kinds of manufacturing plants, control of air conditioning and fire precautions in buildings are some examples of areas which now rely heavily on computerised process control.

In the design of process control systems a long list of deterministic rules is the only major ingredient. The demand on intelligence is not all that significant. Nevertheless, such systems do make it possible for computers to measure, interpret and often correct almost instantly what might take a human expert days, weeks or even longer. Process control may be defined as showing 'intelligence' in this sense. The system can also lead to a highly intelligent expenditure of energy and minimising of costs. This of course is always a paramount consideration and undoubtedly in a complex process the machine's wisdom can easily outperform the wisdom of the human expert by many orders of magnitude.

The knowledge-based or expert system which makes greater demands on AI concepts than process control is designed to deal with complexity that arises through lack of clear deterministic data. Such systems deal in probabilities and not in hard facts. Like process control, these also rely on long lists of rules (typically about 300), but the rules now take the form "If A is likely and B is also likely but C is less likely and D is not the case then E is probably true ". The total number of such rules in a system is called its 'knowledge base' and the expert system operates by drawing inferences from it.

The procedure for 'consultation' with an expert system is rather similar to the one adopted by a human consultant. The consultation begins with a list of questions to build a database for the knowledge base to act on. The end product of a consultation is a list of likelihoods or probabilitites.

It has been demonstrated that there can be many advantages in making such expertise available on a computer. Experts are expensive and the economic benefits of employing an expert system can be very substantial. In such activities as drilling for oil or assessing the suitability of a site for mineral exploitation, the cost of failure can run to hundreds of thousands of pounds per day. Expert systems are increasingly becoming an integral part of most such operations.

Experts are also scarce. The constant availability of expert advice on tap eliminates the need to wait for the expert to become available. It releases the expert's valuable time for tackling more urgent problems.

Human experts have prejudices and failings. They are often overworked and fatigued. Expert systems can help eliminate individual bias, prejudices and errors that frequently result from oversight and fatigue. They can allow for the pooling of knowledge from the best practitioners in the field and thereby evolve into being the finest repository of the state-of-the-art knowledge.

Finally, there is a facility often built into expert systems which makes them ideal tools for teaching. This provides the rationale behind some question, advice or conclusion. The novice can make use of the facility to observe and question the reasoning process of an expert and learn to do the same.

The Future

We have now completed our survey of current developments. We shall close this chapter with a brief vision of the future.

As described earlier, the 'First Generation' computers were built out of valves, the 'Second Generation' out of transistors and the 'Third Generation' used integrated circuits. Todays computers are known as the 'Fourth Generation' machines, characterised by vastly enhanced levels of circuitry packed on integrated circuit chips. The Fourth Generation machines are faster, smaller, cheaper and more interlinked than the previous ones. They have better operating systems, superior programming languages and they employ a more extensive range of algorithms. However, despite order of magnitude gains in all these attributes there has been no radical jump in computer architecture or the way information is organised in a computer.

Whereas gains on the faster-smaller-cheaper-interlinked fronts will undoubtedly continue in the forseeable future, great research effort is now being spent in trying to develop something radically new - to be called the 'Fifth Generation'. These machines were initially planned to appear in the 1990s but the signs are that this expectation was too optimistic.

The Fifth Generation

The object here is to make machines that have the capacity for learning, for recognising patterns, for associating ideas and for drawing inferences from suitably stored knowledge - in other words, machines that display the characteristics of the human brain. The Japanese have coined the term KIPS (Knowledge Information Processing Systems) to describe the projected breed.

The Fifth Generation machines are also to be much more user-friendly than anything we know today. They are expected to be able to read script, recognise voice and faces, synthesize speech, process language, converse in several languages and use everyday methods of communication such as telephone and TV. These are tall orders indeed and there is long way to go, but there are many promising developments.

The concepts enunciated in defining the Fifth Generation machines have also helped to focus the mind on where the computer is going ultimately. It is becoming clear that the computer is in fact a first rudimentary effort of intelligent life on Earth to create a device that functions increasingly like itself. Scientists from a wide range of disciplines such as neural science, psychology, biotechnology, physics and chemistry are joining forces with computer scientists to try to understand and duplicate the functioning of the human brain.

There are other perfectly sober scientists, in receipt of government grants, whose stated ultimate objective is nothing less fantastic than to assemble fully operational computers inside living cells. These researchers are developing bio-chips that work with electro-chemistry rather than just electricity. Their work ultimately promises to bring about chips that are a billion times smaller and a billion times more powerful than the silicon chip. When this promise is realised we will be able to build living computers. Thus the computer, it is clear, is ultimately destined to be the spearhead of future human evolution and as such we can hardly fail to be fascinated by it.

References & Suggestions for Further Reading

1. Fenichel, R. and Weizenbaum, J., "Computers and Computation", Readings from Scientific American, Freeman, 1971. *A good source of historical perspective by many of the early pioneers of computing.*

2. Toong, H. D. and Gupta, A., "Personal Computers", Scientific American, Dec. 1982. *An integrated account of computer hardware and software for the general reader.*

3. "Computer Software ", Scientific American, Sept 1984. *This whole issue is devoted to software by leading practitioners of the art. Suitable for the non-specialist reader.*

4. Feigenbaum, E., and McCorduck, P., "The Fifth Generation", Pan Books, 1984. *Rather a political book. Sets out to rouse America to Japanese challenge. Good thumping Journalism.*

5. Michie, D. and Johnston, R., "The Creative Computer ", Pelican Books, 1984. *Michie who has done most of his work at the Machine Intelligence Unit of Edinburgh University in U.K. (now at Glasgow University) is a pioneer and world renowned figure in AI. The book presents all the major successes of AI so far.*

6. Moto-oka, T. and Kitsuregawa, M. "The Fifth Generation Computer", Wiley, 1985. *Moto-oka is the leader of Japan's Fifth Generation programme. Here with a young colleague he narrates the story of the birth of the Fifth Generation.*

7. Edited by Hayes, J.E. and Michie, D., "Intelligent Systems, The Unprecedented Opportunity", Ellis Harwood, 1984. *Describes knowledge-based systems. A number of leading British and American futurists assess the impact of AI on tomorrow's world.*

8. Dreyfus, H., "What Computers Can't Do : A Critique of Artificial Reason", Harper & Row 1971. *Dreyfus brothers are the leading voices who hold AI in contempt. They have many sober and justifiable things to say but... well, we*

9. Dreyfus, H. and Dreyfus, S., "Mind Over Machine", Free Press (distributed in U.K. by Macmillan Distribution) 1985.
10. Abu-Mostafa, Y. and Psaltis, D., "Optical Neural Computers", Scientific American, March 1987. *Optical technology which promises much faster and more extensively connected (like the brain cells) processing is perhaps the most promising technology for the planned Fifth Generation machines. Two of the leading researchers in the field describe this emerging field.*

3. Computers and the Health of Society

> The Health of the People is the Highest Law.
> (From the 12 Law Tables of Rome)

Everything is ultimately driven by the needs of self-preservation. Every personal or social enterprise can be thought of as being bound up with health. Farming, religion, education, tourism, entertainment, disposal of rubbish and anything else we care to name is connected with the health of society. In this chapter we look at the impact of computers in developing and maintaining the health of society. Clearly, we have to constrain our definition of health-related enterprises in order to be able to focus on some manageable aspect of the whole. We shall restrict ourselves to describing the role of computers in the context of medicine, environment and sport.

Through opening up entirely new possibilities, the computer is rapidly transforming the functioning of many long established institutions. It is also bringing into existence new institutions for tackling problems that could not be tackled before. Such processes are at work, for example, in the administration of patients in hospitals, in the care of the severely handicapped, in the coaching of Olympic athletes and in the devising of new strategies for the management of water resources in the harshest landscapes on earth. In this chapter we shall look at a number of key roles being played by the computer in various areas of health.

Computers in Medicine

Computers deal with medical information in its widest sense, information needed by researchers, drug companies, doctors, nurses, ambulence staff, dieticians, laundry ladies, administrators and of course the patients. The National Health Service in Britain alone is currently spending £100 million a year on computers. In many types of applications, e.g. in the pathology laboratory, computers have been in widespread use for some time. In some other activities such as Patient Administration Systems they are being tried out as something new and there are many other areas such as the exchange of information between primary and secondary care where the matter is largely in research stage. We begin this chapter by examining how computerised tools are providing new ways of diagnosing disease.

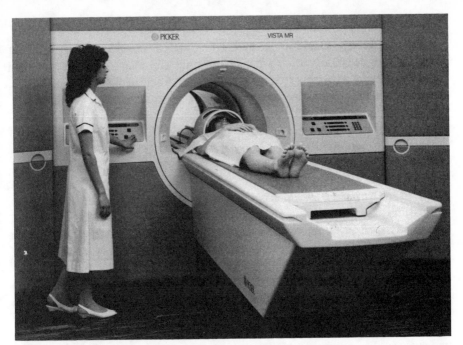

Fig 3.1.   Picker Vista 2055 HP. Magnetic Resonance Imaging System.

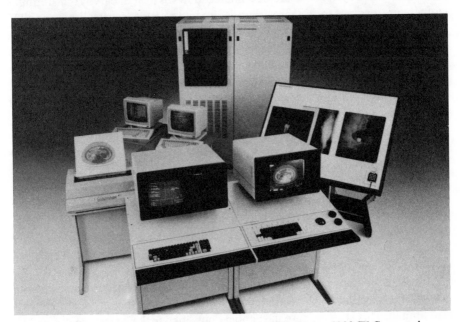

Fig 3.2.   'Synerplan' Therapy Planning System used with the Picker 1200 SX Computed Tomography Scanner.

39

Imaging

The first act of any scientific endeavour that tries to connect cause and effect demands accurate observation. The human senses are of course severely limited and allow only for very restricted observations. To be able to observe more acutely, or to observe phenomena inaccessible to our senses, we continually build new instruments and refine the old ones. For instance, astronomers first relied on optical telescopes of limited power. Then much bigger optical instruments were built, and more recently radio and X-ray telescopes have been added, and so the process goes on.

All acts of observation involve two elements - a *stimulus* from the region to be observed and a *transducer,* which is something that can transform the stimulus into a signal that the human brain can interpret. In the ordinary act of seeing, the reflected or emitted light from an object serves as the stimulus and the cells of the retina acts as the transducers, transforming light into tiny electric currents in the optical nerves.

With the aid of the computer it becomes possible to utilise many other forms of "light" which produce no seeing response in the human eye. This is so because the computer can transform coded signals from any form of transducer whatsoever to turn them into images, sounds or something else that the brain can at once understand. For example, although our eyes are not sensitive to the infra-red radiation emitted by hot bodies, the computer allows us to 'see heat', by transforming temperature readings from a measuring device into colour codes for display on a TV screen or a plotter.

The usefulness of the computer for imaging does not arise merely through its capacity to act as a transducer and relate values from one kind of quantity to values for another. It comes even more so from its power to process these values at great speeds. It can, for example, take thousands of one-dimensional X-ray scans and combine them mathematically to deliver a crisp three dimensional image. If need be, it can then process the image, enlarging, highlighting, rotating, removing unwanted information, and so on. By colouring the picture it can highlight that which might be buried in a smudgy patch of gray.

Through these capabilities of the computer it has become possible to use ultrasound, infrared rays, radio and microwaves, X-rays, magnetic fields and particle beams to see the heart, brain, lungs and other body organs in action inside the body without cutting the body open. The diagnostician is now being offered ever increasing facility to pin-point what is significant and be relieved of that which is of no consequence.

Most of the computerised imaging tools, which we describe in the next section are not yet widely available. The availability of colour and three dimensional pictures is also limited. This is so because the applications often make extensive demand on specialist hardware, computer memory and processing power. However, technology is rapidly overcoming these problems. As we progress in the future the probing of the body through such imaging tools to discover the first signs of disease will become more and more a routine procedure.

Computer tomography (CT scanning)

Before the advent of the computer the need to see inside the body was met for many decades by X-ray radiography. The standard X-ray method, however, has a number of severe limitations. It cannot, for example, discriminate between overlapping structures. It is a one-off activity. Once the picture has been produced its quality cannot be improved. It cannot be viewed from a different perspective without a re-take.

These deficiencies have been overcome with the development of computerised tomography (CT, also called Computer Axial Tomography or CAT). In CT, a series of X-ray scans are recorded from several directions and stored for processing by a computer. This data is combined mathematically by the computer to yield cross-sectional images or slices of the observed region which can be viewed from any perspective. CT gives a much better contrast compared to conventional X-rays and is now a fairly extensively used diagnostic tool in medicine.

Digital subtraction angiography

X-ray penetration depends on the density of tissue and though highly suited to furnishing anatomical information, does not show up soft tissue such as that comprising blood vessels. Information about blood vessels is of vital importance in many kinds of diagnoses, particularly the kind leading to surgery for damaged, blocked, or narrowed arteries.

A method that combines the use of X-rays and contrast agents, which are substances relatively opaque to X-rays, to show what is happening in blood vessels is known as angiography. In this method, an ordinary X-ray scan is first taken, which does not show soft tissue. Next a non-poisonous contrast agent which shows up under X-rays is injected into the patient's blood stream and another X-ray scan taken. Subtracting the unwanted information recorded by the first X-ray from that recorded by the second one produces an image of the blood vessels for diagnosis.

Angiography is more than a tool for diagnosis. Doctors use it to manipulate a tube inside an artery for purposes such as inserting a coil to stop internal bleeding. Many people who would once have bled to death can now be saved with the aid of angiography.

Previously the subtraction process used to be carried out photographically by laboriously superimposing the two negatives together. More recently the process has been speeded up by converting the image to digital information and digital subtraction angiography in now routinely and widely used. However, the images that have been produced have so far remained two-dimensional and rather blurred. They demand considerable skill and judgement for interpretation.

Microcomputer based system are now being developed to turn angiography images into clear 3-D shapes which will make it possible to view them from any perspective and under any sort of illumination. Apart from visual improvement, computerised techniques are also expected to be able to provide accurate quantitative information on the extent and position of damage to blood vessels and also the rate of blood flow through them.

The kind of information will be of very great value in the fight against strokes and ischaemic heart disease - the narrowing and blocking of arteries that supply blood to the muscles of the heart - which together account for the largest numbers of deaths in the Western world. A microcomputer-based system would also be cheap and therefore affordable by more than just a handful of hospitals, where such diagnosis is at present carried out.

Radio isotope methods

The introduction of a small amount of radioactive substance into the body to act as an emitter, utilising the computer to produce an image, has a number of variations and can be tailored to suit special requirements. Procedures of this kind are widely used in the detection of tumours, for example.

Some radiopharmaceuticals have the property of concentrating in malignant tumours, so that after the administration of such substances the region of the tumour emits more radioactivity than the surrouding tissue. A device called a *Gamma Camera,* which is a radiation detector tuned to the particular radiation being emitted, is used to pinpoint the region of radioactivity and a computer is again used to assemble the picture.

Experience gained with diagnostics using radioactive materials is currently being utilised to try to develop a class of drugs with very specific effects. Because these drugs will have very few side effects they are sometimes called 'magic bullets'. These drugs will contain specially engineered molecules (discussed later) that will carry a high dose of radioactivity. The molecules will home in very precisely on malignant sites and destroy the tumours with their radioactivity. This is currently one of the major hopes of some researchers involved in the fight against cancer.

Positron emission tomography (PET)

X-rays, as explained earlier, rely on tissue density differences and therefore cannot yield functional or physiological information since these activities do not give rise to any significant changes in density.

Positron emission tomography (PET) is a powerful non-invasive method for observing changes in metabolic activity in the brain and also in other organs of the body. It exploits the fact that an increase in metabolic activity in a region leads to an increased blood flow in that region as those cells increase their demand for nutrients.

For a PET scan the subject swallows, inhales, or is injected with a small amount of radioactive nutrient. The radioactivity is short-lived and decays rapidly through the emission of subatomic particles called positrons, hence the name. The flow of radioactive nutrients is observed by a PET scanner in the way that one might observe a number of persons with candles moving around at night in a dark house. The radioactivity is revealed by the positrons being radiated away.

PET has proved particularly useful in understanding normal brain function. It has been used, for example, in identifying specific areas of the brain associated with various types of activities such as listening to music, doing mental arithmetic, opening and closing the eyes, raising and lowering of the arms. These actions cause local changes in blood flow as the nutrient uptake increases. This gives rise to changes in radioactive concentrations (positron hot spots). These are detected and fed to the computer as thousands of separate measurements, and exactly as in CT, the computer processes this information to produce an integrated image.

PET is being used not only by neuroscientists but also by many other clinical investigators. Strokes, brain tumours, dementia, schizophrenia, depression are examples of clinical topics currently being aided through the use of PET.

PET is an expensive tool. The radioisotopes used in PET imaging are produced in a machine called the cylotron and have short active lives of the order of a few tens of minutes. This means that the imaging has to be done close to a cyclotron site and the technique demands the collaboration of a team of highly skilled professionals. At present only a small number of places are equipped to offer PET.

Nuclear magnetic resonance (NMR)

In 1979 scientists at the British electronics company EMI produced the first pictures of the human brain utilising an effect known in atomic physics as nuclear magnetic resonance (NMR). NMR provides information about chemical composition at the cellular level and is a powerful new diagnostic tool in medicine for discriminating accurately between healthy and diseased cells. NMR can reveal the extent of cancers and assess brain damage, muscular distrophy and heart disease. The

43

suitability of organs for transplants can be ascertained, and indeed NMR can be used in any other investigation of cellular damage.

NMR shows up structures which X-rays cannot reveal, and has the advantage of not exposing the subject to the kind of ionising radiation used in CT. Although minute, this nevertheless carries a slight risk of damage to healthy tissue.

A simplified description of the way NMR operates is as follows. The nuclei of most atoms behave like tiny magnets. If an oscillating magnetic field of the right frequency is applied, then a specific population of nuclei resonates with the field and absorbs energy. When the field is switched off, then the same nuclei emit the absorbed energy and from this their positions can be inferred. The frequencies used in NMR are radio frequencies and do not cause tissue damage.

The interpretation of NMR requires a knowledge of the chemical differences which exist between damaged and healthy tissue. It is known, for example, that the distribution of water molecules is often altered in diseased tissues. By tuning in to the nuclei of these molecules, NMR is able to show accurately the distribution of water and hence the extent of the diseased cells.

Once again, NMR relies on the computer to assemble the pictures and deliver them as meaningful images.

Ultrasonography

This method uses high frequency sound waves of several million cycles per second to create echoes in the way a ship's sonar does in charting the ocean floor. The echoes are fed into a computer which processes them as in other methods described above. Ultrasonography is highly accurate and can show different types of tissue which are not revealed by normal X-ray studies. Ultrasound equipment is also much less costly and like NMR, carries no risk from radiation.

Ultrasound is heavily used in obstetrics where it is used to monitor the development of a foetus and diagnose complications in childbirth and pregnancy. In Britain, for example, four out of five pregnant women receive ultrasound observation.

Thermal imaging

CT, PET, NMR and ultrasound are all used for observing structures inside the body. One computer-based technique for observing the surface of the body is based on thermal imaging or thermography.

Human eyes are only sensitive to that small range of frequencies embedded in the full spectrum that pervades the environment, called light. Heat radiation differs from light only in its frequency but humans are blind to it just as they are deaf to certain frequencies that a dog can hear.

By interfacing heat detecting sensors with the computer, thermography makes visible temperature patterns which are normally invisible. We can then see the ebb and flow of temperature changes when, for example, a person becomes stressed and then relaxes. Some diseases, such as breast cancer, produce local hot spots, and for such diseases thermography is a valuable tool of diagnosis.

Apart from its diagnostic value, thermography yields images that are fascinating, rich and complex and almost worthy of being regarded as an art form.

Other Examples of Computerised Diagnostics

Detection of cell abnormalities

In all the examples given previously the basic role of the computer involves image processing. The techniques described above are fairly well established. There are many new areas involving computerised image analysis that are currently being developed. We will mention one such example from the pathology laboratory where the computer is already well established for many types of analysis on many types of bodily specimens.

Several groups are trying to develop computerised techniques for automatic or interactive detection of cell abnormalities. Typically, in this application a computer scans sets of microscope-produced slides containing images of cells. Abnormal cells or foreign bodies normally have different shapes and densities compared to the healthy ones and are picked up and recorded by the computer. These can then be examined interactively by the diagnostician. In this way a very large number of cell samples can be processed. This kind of automation will be a major factor in making feasible the screening of very large populations.

Signal processing

Another well established area of diagnostic use is in the processing of electrical and other physiological signals from organs such as the heart, brain and lungs.

In many clinical situations, such as surgery, intensive care and high-risk pregnancy, the subject needs to be diagnosed continuously or at least fairly regularly over a long period and responded to immediately should the need arise.

The computer is an ideal tool for keeping a sensitive and detailed watch in all such situations. Readings of pulse rate, heart and brain waveforms, respiration rate, volume of air breathed, blood pressure, foetal heart rate and blood sugar levels are examples of important diagnostics that can all be provided accurately, conveniently and at high speed. The instantaneous displays of these signals and also their statistical summaries provided by a computer are now routinely used in many clinical situations. Without the use of the computer such readings demand a whole army of specialists and even then are slow, and error prone. They are also much more costly.

The computer can not only observe but can also take a variety of appropriate actions. In particular it can ring an alarm to alert the appropriate person and it can advise the clinician by providing him with rapid access to information.

Sophisticated diagnostics for the GP

Thanks to the cheapness and portability of microcomputers, the kind of diagnostic facilities which have previously been available only at hospitals or at specialist laboratories are more and more likely to become available at the family doctor level.

An example of a development in this direction is the launch of a computerised screening machine in May 1987 by the British company, Medical Universal. The machine has been designed with the help of scientists from Brunel University and has been claimed as being the most advanced health screening unit of its kind in the world. It checks the functioning of the heart and lungs and analyses blood chemistry and can rapidly point out signs of abnormalities in such things as blood pressure, liver and kidney function and respiratory function. The machine is operated by a technician and only requires about ten minutes or so of the doctor's attention for the final interpretation.

It will be able to carry out early detection of heart disease, bronchitis, diabetes, blood disorders, industrial diseases and many other afflictions which at present are often able to progress far before being noticed.

Diagnosing ear disease

Another diagnostic tool developed at Brunel University is the Tympanic Membrane Displacement System (TMD) for accurate detection of diseases of the middle and inner ear.

Minute changes in movements of the eardrum can reveal disorders inside the ear and can also point to tumours or other malfunctioning in the parts of the brain concerned with hearing. The TMD apparatus plays a repeated note through an earphone worn by the patient and the resulting movement of the eardrum is conveyed via a diaphragm to a computer. The movement is displayed by the computer on a monitor and from this any abnormalities can be readily picked up by the specialist. TMD analysis takes only two to three minutes and does not involve any discomfort for the patient.

Diagnosis at a distance

The time and effort spent in travelling to a specialist is wasteful and particularly so if the diagnosis is negative. Ideally the specialist should travel to the patient.

On-line monitoring relieves the specialist of the need to be physically close to the patient. This makes for easier and better care and can also lead to significant cost reductions. Such is the case, for example, of the system developed for monitoring foetal heart rates in high-risk pregnancies by Dr. Kevin Dalton, consultant in obstetrics and gynechology at Cambridge, U.K., in collaboration with Dr. Michael Bright, consultant obstetrician at Rosie Maternity Hospital. There system, christened the Cambridge Telemetry System, provides pregnant women with a portable ultrasonic foetal heart monitor which can be linked to a computer via an ordinary telephone. The expectant mothers phone in a recording of their baby's heart to the hospital once a day over the telephone-computer link for analysis.

In this way the women receive regular monitoring without having to travel long distances two or three times a week and be kept waiting in hospital. They need only be admitted if something abnormal is detected, which the computer can pick up with great rapidity.

The procedure is not only more efficient and more convenient but results in substantial savings. Without on-line monitoring being available, some of these women would have to occupy a bed in hospital costing £150 or so per day. Compared to that the cost of a twenty minute cheap rate phone call is insignificant.

This kind of monitoring will undoubtedly become a more common mode of observation for many clinical situations where todays methods are tedious and costly.

Knowledge-based systems in medicine

In chapter 2 we described the general concept of an expert or knowledge-based system. This is a tool for dealing with complex situations and relies on a large data base comprising a set of rules such as 'If A is true and B is true then X is true', or, 'If A is true and B is true then there is a seventy percent probability that X is true.'

Medical diagnosis, even for apparently simple complaints, can be highly complex. Consider the case of acute abdominal pain as an example. It could result from appendicitis, pancreatitis, food poisioning, displaced foetus in pregnancy, and from a multitude of other causes.

Medical diagnosis is essentially rule-based. The clinician basically folows a set of rules - ' If the patients has a runny nose and a high temperature then it is probable that.....' For this reason the sphere of medicine, particularly in U.S.A, has given rise to a large number of successful expert systems.

One of the earliest and most publicised ones is MYCIN, developed at Stanford University in the mid-1970s for diagnosing and prescribing antibiotic treatment for bacterial infections such as meningitis. The system is based on a large set of *knowledge rules* from which the probability of any given diagnosis being correct can be calculated, given the patients symptoms.

The diagnosis is arrived at as a result of a question and answer dialogue between the computer and the doctor. The patient's symptoms, signs and other information are thus interpreted in the light of the expert system rules. Most questions are in a form requiring only a YES and NO response and an important feature of the system is that by typing 'RULE' or 'WHY' the doctor can observe which rules are being applied in the processing, and obtain the reasons behind a diagnosis. This feature allays fears and suspicion and the doctor, if unimpressed by the answers, can act readily to overrule the computer's judgement.

Thus the expert system approach is intended to help the doctor and not to replace him. The facility for being able to obtain explanations at each step is clearly of high educational value and may be used for the training of students in the art and science of diagnosis.

MYCIN helped enormously in gaining acceptance for expert systems in medicine by demonstrating repeatedly that not only could it perform on a par with human experts, but often outdo them. In one test ten difficult cases were selected. Nine doctors were supplied with details of the symptoms and MYCIN was also given a trial. The diagnoses produced by the doctors, together with the one produced by the computer, were presented to specialists for evaluation. MYCIN achieved the highest score. Many such tests have now firmly established the credibility of expert systems.

Since the advent of MYCIN many more exert systems have been developed in the field. For example, ONCOCIN plans drug therapy for cancer patients, HEADMEAD prescribes antipsychotic drugs for mental patients, PUFF diagnoses lung disease. In the U.S. access to all these is available on a network called SUMEX-AM (Stanford University Medical Experimental Computer for Artificial Intelligence in Medicine). The network is part of a government-funded project which links terminals in medical centres to the main computer housed at Rutgers University in California.

Whereas the U.S. has so far produced the most publicised of expert systems in medicine, significant work is being done in many other countries. In the U.K., for example, the computer manufacturers ICL have recently announced an expert system to help in the diagnosis of acute abdominal pain. The system can consult a database of 10000 cases collected worldwide with the help of the World Organisation of Gastroenterology, based on the work of Dr. de Dombal, a Reader in Clinical Information Science in the Department of Surgery at the University of Leeds. It has been estimated that if exploited on a national basis de Dombal's system could save the British National Health Service more than £20 million annually.

Although most expert systems are at present limited to diagnosing one type of disease, there are some that cover a wider range. Such a system is CADUCEUS developed by Dr. Jack Myers and his colleagues at the University of Pittsburgh School of Medicine in U.S.A. It has a database of about 4000 symptoms associated with more than 500 ailments. CADUCEUS has demonstrated the reliability of a general purpose expert system as MYCIN did for specialist ones. In tests CADUCEUS successfuly diagnosed straightforward 'textbook' symptoms in mere thirty seconds, and has 'passed' the examination of the American Board of Internal Medicine which certifies medical specialists.

Although there has to be much more research before expert systems in medicine come into wide-scale usage, it has been convincingly deemonstrated that their promise is considerable. As developments in Artificial Intelligence proceed, expert systems in medicine will become increasingly sophisticated. They will, by collecting data from all over the world and expertise from leading specialists, deliver better and cheaper health care than is on offer today. No single individual can be expected to carry all the current knowledge in his head and expert systems will undoubtedly become essential decision support aids for all specialists.

Computers for sharing of medical information

Despite the fact that a doctor in the U.K. is obliged to report contraindications about a patient when the patient is referred to a hospital for treatment, it is estimated that about 300 patients die each year under anaesthesia, many of these deaths being caused by adverse reactions peculiar to a patient. This is just one example of a situation where vital medical information is not exchanged effectively and rapidly enough. It also highlights the fact that in an emergency a practioner, in this case the anaesthetist, needs to make rapid decisions about an uncommon occurance. This demands instant access to expert advice.

The reasons for failures in medical information exchange are easy to appreciate. Medical records are frequently bulky and may typically involve 20 to 30 sheets of paper. Medical care is divided into primary care at the family doctor and secondary care at a variety of hospitals. The various specialist groups in a hospital are all fragmented, disparate and housed in different locations. A large hospital may well be involved in the processing of tens of thousand of patient records at a time and so on.

Thus although information ought ideally to be available when it is needed and where it is needed, it is easy to appreciate that the extraction and presentation of medical information at the right place and at the right time is in general a daunting task.

Not surprisingly, computers of all kinds, from huge mainframes to hand held micros, are revolutionising the traditional methods of medical information exchange. There are many problems, e.g. the need for confidentiality, standardisation of methods of recording data, standardisation of computer hardware and software, etc. but undoubtedly this is a major area of application and rapid developments are taking place in many areas.

Going back to the problem faced by anaesthetists with which we opened this section, the National Adverse Reaction Drug Advisory Service in the U.K. has unveiled plans to equip U.K. hospitals with small portable microcomputers which will provide anaesthetists with on-the-spot expert advice in cases of adverse drug reaction.

In U.K. the Community Health Information Project (CHIP) is exploring the development of networks for information exchange between the GP, the health authority and the family practitioner committee. In Japan the Medical Systems Development Centre in Tokyo has been involved for some years in developing information systems. Local networks are being created and regional centres are being linked to urban centres. In some places in Japan the patient now arrives at the outpatient department of a hospital carrying a plastic card similar to an ordinary credit card. Within ten minutes or so the patient is called up to see the doctor who by then has all the relevant information and records, ready on his desk top. The Welsh School of Pharmacy have devised a similar card, called the Smart Card for the sharing of information between a GP and a pharmacist.

The major effort in the sharing of information is intended to bring about the situation where all the different hospitals, units and consulting rooms in primary and secondary care are all networked together. Terminals in pathology, pharmacy, accident and emergency units, laundry room and the clinic run by the family doctor will all be able to record, transmit and receive information via the network. Picture Archiving Communication Systems (PACS) currently under development will allow the transmission of patient's X-ray pictures and other diagnostic images. The state of the art expert knowledge on any speciality and also complete ongoing health profiles of individuals will become available at all points in the network. The appropriate portion of this information will be immediately accessible to any properly authorised user.

Typically, the family doctor will use the network to record and transmit information about the history of disease in a patient, his family history and any idiosyncratic reactions. This information will be directly available for diagnostics at the hospital. The hospital will in turn do the same regarding the outcome of a patient's visit, his diagnostics such as X-rays, pathalogy reports, condition on discharge and recommendations for treatment. This information will reach the GP immediately. The handling of such items as waiting lists for operations, and appointments to see consultants, etc. will all be done interactively. The GP will play a much bigger role in the mangement of such two-way activities than has been possible in the past.

The network will allow expert knowledge to be shared between different specialists, departments, districts, regions and nations. It will also allow restricted access to manufacturers and vendors of drugs, medical equipment and other support services. For example, the GP's prescription will be promptly transmitted to the local chemist for preparation.

Implicit in this mode of handling health information is the ease of collection of health statistics and the possibility for better resource management, evaluation of performance and prevention. At present statistics are collected laboriously and a vast amount of potentially useful information remains untapped. For example, around 90% of events of ill health are handled by the GP but are recorded mostly in structureless and illegible scrawls. This information could give all sorts of insights regarding the local environment, both physical and social, and the effect of changes in it. The medium and the format of recording, however, keeps these insights buried and inaccessible. The result is much duplication of effort, waste and imbalanced deployment of resources.

We shall now look at two examples of important developments in information sharing.

Patient administration systems (PAS)

Over the last few years most major hospitals in advanced countries have begun to deploy PAS to support and administer their activities. One of the major international suppliers in this field is the American company Mcdonnell Douglas Information Systems and we shall describe their product to explain the function of PAS.

The Mcdonnell Douglas system comprises about a dozen or so modules. The modules can be installed to work independently as "stand-alone" or as part of an integrated system. The key module around which all other modules are built is the MASTER PATIENT INDEX (MPI).

Clearly, the most basic piece of information that every one needs and that ought to be shared in a health care environment has to do with the personal details of patients. The MPI is designed to do just that. It contains a record of all patients registered at a hospital, whether they are currently admitted or not. It allows for very comprehensive information to be held on each patient: names and aliases, present and several preceding addresses, date of birth, sex, marital status, religion, nationality, identity information, e.g. National Insurance Number in Britain, languages spoken, etc. Each patient record is associated with a Case Record Number.

The MPI acts as a central reference file to be shared by all modules of the total system. It can be accessed by any authorised user within any department of the hospital or in any other hospital that shares a linked network. The MPI cuts out a great deal of tedious, repetitious and error prone form filling that has to be done otherwise. It offers the user the advantage of taking him swiftly to a single record that he is after instead of a the mountains of files that usually have to be sifted.

A second key module is known as INPATIENTS. This module provides access to information on admission details; the date, source, type of admission; the speciality and ward to which the patient has been assigned; emergency contacts of the patient and so on. It maintains current information on transfers between wards and consultants; the numbers of empty and occupied beds in various wards, etc.

In common with all other modules the INPATIENTS module minimises paperwork. Its key function is, however, to optimise bed use. The instant access to bed occupancy information means that a bed can be utilised as soon as the patient occupying it has been discharged. Without such an aid it can take several hours to gather the information and sorely needed beds often remain unoccupied. The module serves the key overall function of providing statistical information for management on bed occupancy. Such information is vital for future planning and for optimum deployment of resources.

There are a dozen or so such modules in a PAS. Other modules handle information about outpatients, waiting lists, accident and emergency, maternity and obstetrics, birth registrations, theatre bookings and so on. In an even more integrated approach the modules of the PAS interface with modules from other units. For example, the CLINICAL SERVICES modules allow for checks to be made with laboratories regarding drug therapy associated with a particular patient; OPERATIONAL SERVICES modules yield information relating to the availability of ambulances and so on.

Sharing of information on poisoning

The technological society produces an ever increasing number and variety of toxic substances for industrial, agricultural and medicinal use. Consequently, there is a steady increase in out of the ordinary cases of poisoning reported to GPs and hospitals. No one can be expected to have an up-to-date knowledge of all the toxic materials that are in existence at any stage and yet it is essential that the medical practitioner who is called to attend should respond rapidly.

There could hardly be a more pressing case for the sharing of medical information and not surprisingly Poisons Informations Services began to come into existence in developed countries from as long ago as 1949, having first been established in the Netherlands. Their major aim is to provide a 24 hour emergency service to doctors for the diagnosis and treatment of serious or unusual cases of poisoning but, as for the PAS, they are also able to provide essential statistical insights for management. These services rely increasingly on computerised databases, expert systems, and electronic information sharing procedures using networks.

Such, for example, is the service provided by the Viewdata Project of the Scottish Poisons Information Bureau located in Edinburgh, U.K. The project maintains an up-to-date database on poisons which is continually revised. The Bureau provides rapid expert advice to the medical profession and also supplies literature on facilities such as addresses of laboratories where poisons can be analyzed.

Computers in the education of doctors and patients

As we saw earlier, expert systems provide a new way of teaching trainee doctors and indeed other medical personnel such as nurses and ambulance staff. Everyone has heard that a picture is worth a thousand words and it is through the exploitation of computer graphics that it becomes possible to develop truly efficient methods of teaching. Such methods, as we shall see, are also relevant for the education of the patient, something which has so far been completely ignored.

The constraints of teaching anatomy from a book or physiology from a corpse are pretty obvious. Ideally the student needs a three dimensional model which can be made to respond structurally and functionally in exactly the way that a real body would, revealing all the relevant details that need to be learnt. Such a model is also potentially of very great value to patients, for it is widely recognised that they often experience a great deal of unnecessary worry through the ignorance of the workings of their own bodies. It would be very comforting, for example, to be able to explain easily what a gall bladder operation or a kidney stone removal involves.

With the growth of litigation, particularly in the USA, this need has grown and doctors are increasingly expected to try and inform their patients as fully as possible about the risks associated with any proposed course of treatment. Self respect also demands that consent to treatment should be based on information rather than mere acquiscence. Computer graphics is making it possible to satisfy these needs of the doctor and the patient.

One of the great pioneers of computer graphics in general medical education is Professor Chuck Csuri, head of Ohio State University's Department of Art Education at Columbus, U.S.A., whose company Cranston-Csuri Productions has develped a spectacular 3-D computer animation method for showing the functioning of the internal organs of the human body. One can watch from any angle the simulated action of the heart, lungs and other major organs. The shapes and colours of the images mimic very precisely those of the real organs.

Another development in computer graphics that is relevant for the training of surgeons has come from the work of Dr. Donald Meacher of Phoenix Data Systems in Albany, New York. He has developed a powerful new method for organising data in computer memory on images of three dimensional objects. His method makes it possible for a particular view of the stored image to be produced very rapidly.

The 3-D images that are produced are constructed from a set of 2-D images which themselves are extracted from CT scans or some other imaging tool of the type described earlier. Typically, about 60 2-D images are used to assemble a complete 3-D image of the brain.

Meacher's method is a true 3-D method in so far as it allows for cut-away views of the object. Thus when a cut is made to simulate an operation the image on the screen splits into two and two images appear to show the structures that lie on either side of the incision. Meacher's method makes it possible to do for surgery what flight simulators have done for the training of pilots. Medical students will be able to practice incisions or complete operations as often as they like and without any risk to patients or to themselves exactly as trainee pilots are able to practice flying manoeuvres without any risk to passengers, aeroplanes or themselves.

Modelling

The scientific use of the term 'modelling' needs to be explained. Suppose that aeroplanes had not been invented and one suddenly felt the urge to design a craft that could fly. Developments might take place as follows. Initally a number of toy models are built to predict how the real craft should behave. These experiments then lead to an actual full size craft. The craft may behave reasonably as expected or it may be an utter disaster.

The making of actual physical models, vital though it often is in the initial stages, is of limited use because it is time consuming and cannot cater for all possible variations. Experience with physical models leads to the understanding of principles which can be stated in mathematical terms and real predictive power comes from mathematical models. In the case of our flying machine, the principles involved are the laws of aerodynamics, and 'modelling' simply means working out the consequences of these laws in a given situation. The better we understand the laws of aerodynamics, the more accurately we can predict the behaviour of aeroplanes from these mathematical 'models' without actually having to physically construct them. The more accurately a mathematical model reflects physical reality, the more complex it is likely to be and so computers are essential to work out its consequences, and this kind of activity is called 'computer modelling'.

Models differ in the range of applicability and need not 'look' anything like the real thing. To predict the orbit of the Earth around the sun we can model them both as 'points' in space. This model would not be able to predict the tides or the phenomena of night and day. Such predictions become possible if we model the Earth as a rotating sphere. In this manner scientists continually refine their models so as to be able to predict a more extensive range of effects.

Computers in molecular biology

We are able to design nuclear reactors and explode hydrogen bombs because physics has provided us with good models of atomic structures and of atomic interactions. The properties of any material, living or non-living, depend entirely on the structures and interactions of molecules. These are assemblies of atoms which represent the smallest chemical unit of that material. Our facility to control and manipulate living organisms depends ultimately on the quality of our molecular models.

In parallel with micro-electronics, micro-biology has also made revolutionary strides in the last few decades through gaining a greatly extended understanding of molecular structures and interactions. Typically, workers at the University of California recently published the structure of an enzyme known as TS down to a resolution of 30 billionth of a centimetre. It is through understanding structures and interactions at this kind of level that it has become possible to do such things as coax bacteria to function as factories for the manufacturing of human insulin for the treatment of diabetis. It is this kind of knowledge that is leading us to disentangle the ultimate basis of life itself.

To continue their advances, biologists need powerful theoretical models which can simulate these processes and computers are at the heart of these simulations. Computers are active in every aspect of modelling but one of their key contributions again springs from making available the facility to visualise three-dimensional molecular structures. The structures that are of interest often involve tens of thousands of atoms and for this reason this enterprise is one of the biggest users of supercomputers.

One class of structures that are of great significance are those of proteins. Protein molecules are fundamental to life and their structures determine most of the physiological behaviour of a living cell. In the form of enzymes they act as catalysts to regulate life's everyday biochemical processes such as food digestion. They are also needed for rarer events, e.g. the male sperm carries an enzyme whose action is essential in enabling the sperm to penetrate the tough outer coating around the female ovum.

Protein molecules are also central in the continuous fight against infections waged by our immune system. The immune system detects potentially harmful foreign substances called antigens which are proteins that form the outer surfaces of bacteria, viruses and other organisms which invade the body. Part of the immune system, the white blood cells or lymphocytes manufactured in the spleen and thymus respond to this invasion by making their own proteins, called antibodies. The antibodies neutralise the antigens rather as a key fits a lock, and it is the structure of the proteins involved that renders the antigens harmless. For these reasons the designers of drugs and vaccines seek to understand the structures of proteins that form antigens and antibodies.

Traditionally, the need to visualise molecular structures has been met by constructing ball and stick models made from wood, metal and plastic. These physical models are cumbursome and inefficient. Even if they represent only a moderately large number of atoms, they take substantial amount of time to build. They occupy large amounts of space and cannot be easily altered. They do not provide easy answers to such questions as "What is the distance between this atom and that one? " In time they become distorted and damaged.

Computer graphics offers a far faster and more effective alternative to building physical molecular models. Computer models of molecules or parts of molecules can be viewed effectively from a variety of perspectives, in various contrast and colours. They can be modified and shaped at will and are not subject to ever increasing errors due to wear and tear or bulk.

For these reasons one very rapidly growing area of computer involvement in biology and indeed the whole of chemistry is that of molecular graphics. This is the science of modelling molecular structures and interactions using computer graphics. Most of the world's major pharmaceutical companies are active in this field and the use of molecular graphics is leading to a revolution in drug design.

Molecular graphics makes it possible to simulate the interactions of drug molecules and their targets. From this knowledge molecules can be engineered to possess properties relevant to a desired application, e.g. specific binding capabilities to tumours. In this way a whole range of new tailor-made anticancer, antimicrobial and other therapeutic drugs are expected to become available.

The new methods of drug design are also providing answers for some old invasive diseases that have refused to go away. The battle against malaria, for example, is now centuries old, yet half the world's population is still at risk and between eight and nine million people die each year from the disease.

In the Sixties it was expected that the battle against malaria would soon be won through a combination of drugs and insecticides. But the mosquito soon began to develop resistence to insecticide and the malarial parasite carried by the mosquito managed to do the same against chloroquine, the anti-malarial drug developed from quinine. In 1959 two countries reported this kind of resistence. By 1980 the number was 26 and in just four more years the number of countries had risen to 40.

It now seems that science will after all be able to tip the balance against malaria again. At an international conference on tropical diseases held in Geneva in June 1986 news of successful trials using new genetically engineered and synthetic vaccines was reported. Such vaccines and other tailor-made drugs to fight scourges such as malaria are becoming possible through the contribution of computers to microbiology.

Computers for the handicapped

Nowhere is the compassionate face of the computer more visible than when offering aids to the handicapped. Many who are crippled, paralysed, deaf, unable to speak and suffer from all sorts of other misfortunes, have become full of life, eager to communicate and remarkably independent - thanks to computers.

As was explained in chapter 2, there is no restriction at all on the kind of input and output interfaces that may be attached to the computer. All that is needed is a transducer to change some consistant action into codes for input to the machine. Examples of consistent actions which are being used by severely handicapped people to drive the computer are: small movements of the head, movements of the pelvis, sucking, blowing, whistling, clapping, eye movement, pressing a single switch with a stick held in the teeth, pressing a couple of switches with the sides of the head and many similar limited actions. These actions are being used as aids to communications and mobility, and in learning and entertainment.

The computer is increasingly offering the handicapped the chance to achieve their potential at work and play in ways that have never been possible. For example, through the use of computers, it has become possible for severely physically handicapped children, such as those with cerebral palsy, to compose and play music and thus be part of the pop culture. Researchers at East Carolina University in the USA have developed a computer system that enables blind chemists to identify chemical compounds by turning spectrometer readings into a series of musical notes, and so on. Great strides are being made on a very extensive front indeed and we shall now describe one project in some detail. The project is picked for being very representative of modern work and thinking in this field.

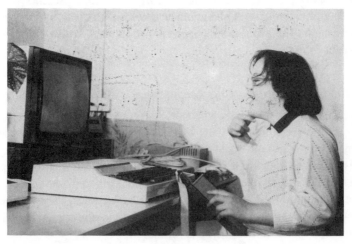

Fig 3.3. A handicapped user at the Royal Earlswood Hospital, UK.

Royal Earlswood Hospital in Redhill, U.K., houses approximately 500 mentally handicapped people with learning difficulties. Many also have physical handicaps such as impaired sight, hearing and speech. The most severely handicapped require total care. The hospital also serves similarly handicapped persons living in their own homes in the East Surrey Health District.

In mid-1986, after some pilot work, the hospital installed a network system using the well known BBC Master microcomputer. The computers are located in key areas of the hospital such as wards and Departments of Psychology, Occupational Therapy, Physiotherapy and Further Education, making a multi-specialist involvement possible.

The directors of the programme have focussed on three ways in which the Computer Network can enhance the quality of life of the handicapped and at the same time contribute to greater scientific understanding of their handicap. The following objectives and expectations of the Computer Network Project at Royal Earlswood Hospital have been supplied to the author by Dr. V. Palmer, Director of Psychological Services of the East Surrey Health Authority in U.K.

1. Communication Skills & Intellectual Development

Many residents have multiple disabilities which make it difficult for them to learn, speak or to use sign language effectively; for these men and women, the microprocessors will offer a new opportunity to communicate their needs, feelings and experiences, either by the use of picture language, or even a written language. For deaf residents it will mean a breakthrough in learning language skills and even for the blind, a system can be adapted so that so that they can experiment with sound effects and easily make up sound pictures of their own. Residents who cannot communicate effectively with one another may learn to do so by joint use of the computer system. The avenues this opens are some of the most exciting that the system has to offer.

2. Independence for the physically handicapped

For a small number of residents, who are so severely handicapped physically that they can do little or nothing for themselves, it is hoped to use microprocessors to give them an opportunity to take an active part in exploration and learning which their physical disabilities have so far denied them. Because it will be possible to adapt the control to allow them to choose programs, and to work independently to produce effects upon the video-screens of their own choice, they will be able to interact with their environment in a new way and thus gain a measure of independence, in spite of their physical limitation.

3. Constructive use of leisure

It is extremely difficult to find a range of materials suitable for the use of residents in their leisure time, the needs of each person are different and everyone grows bored with using the same materials, whether they are toys or books and games. What the computer system can offer is a wide menu of computer games (many of an educational nature) to suit all ability levels. This will allow staff who care for the residents to find suitable material and new material in a matter of minutes for each resident - a task which is normally difficult, expensive and very time consuming. The opportunities for informal learning that this offers are simply great, and the pleasure it will give the resident is important. Because it will be possible to select materials to suit individual needs, it will also provide opportunities for people to experience success, and this is important both in providing motivation for further exploration and enhancing self esteem"

Computers in Environmental Sciences

After the publicity received by such recent catastrophies as the Russian nuclear reactor fire at Chernobyl and the drought-induced mass starvation in Ethiopia, the importance of environmental sciences in safeguarding human health and well-being need hardly be laboured. It is now commonplace to stress that the future of the human species is intertwined with the future of the life-support systems of our environment.

The life-support systems of the environment depend on a multitude of physical and human factors and during the last few decades the range of environmental sciences has grown enormously to cater for studies of these factors. This growth, as one would expect, has relied heavily on the computer. Indeed some of these sciences, such as weather prediction, which involve many processes interacting in complex ways, have only become possible through the availability of the computer.

In what follows the reader should be able to see many parallels between the role of the computer in environmental sciences and its role in medicine described in the last section. For example, the computer makes possible the design of powerful new tools for observing and diagnosing the environment. It offers the sharing of environmental information for operational efficiency and collection of statistical information. It allows prediction and control based on modelling of phenomena. It opens up entirely new ways of helping those who have previously been helpless victims of handicapped environments, for example, the drought-ridden people of Central Africa. Our object in this section is to look at a some examples of methods and applications of computers in these areas.

Diagnosing the environment: Remote Sensing

As in other applications, computers are used in a variety of ways for capturing, storing, transmitting and analyzing environmental data but Remote Sensing represents a particularly spectacular new develpment. This method is unique to environmental sciences and it is therefore appropriate here to look at the principles behind it.

To view an extensive portion of our physical environment, we have to look at it from some height. If we climb a hill we can see more. If we go up in a balloon or an aeroplane our view is enlarged further. This is the simple logic behind the new science of Remote Sensing.

Remote Sensing is the science of obtaining and interpreting information about the Earth's environment from measurements made from some distance from the earth. It began in a small way several decades ago with instruments carried in aeroplanes and balloons, but in the past 20 or so years orbitting satellite technology combined with computerised image analysis has revolutionised the subject.

Instruments of observation carried aboard orbiting satellites are now providing a torrent of information about the Earth from vantage points deep in space. Frequent repetitive coverage of the Earth's surface is revealing information at various scales from local data at resolutions of tens of metres to whole Earth views at several thousand kilometres. We are seeing amazingly detailed and breathtakingly beautiful images of oceans, deserts, lakes, continents, countries, rivers, towns, villages, cloud formations and weather patterns as never been seen before. Some of the remote tracts of our planet situated in the midst of oceans, mountains, deserts and tropical forest are being observed for the first time in human history. Most people have seen a small sample of these, though they may not have heard of Remote Sensing, since images sent by meterological satellites have in the last few years become universal sources of weather forecasts as seen in colour on TV.

The U.S. space programme pioneered the development of Remote Sensing and Landsat-1, launched by NASA in 1972, was the first satellite instrumented specially to collect information about the Earth's surface and its resources. Since then four more Landsats and many other satellites have been launched. Some like the Landsats are placed in near-Earth orbits about 1000 kilometres up and provide regional views of the Earth. Others are much higher up and cover a larger surface. For example, the meteorological satellite Meteosat launched by the European Space Agency, is one of a global network of meteorological satellites occupying a geostationary orbit 36000 kilometres up. Meteosat monitors the complete Earth disc (approximately 1/4 of the Earth's surface) and transmits data every thirty minutes.

The instruments carried by these satellites detect, measure and record selectively filtered radiation. Different features in the environment radiate and absorb different frequencies of radiation and by filtering out some and recording the others, these observations pick out features such as cloud cover, vegetation, temperatures or can take ordinary photographs through the use of the visible frequencies of light.

Most of the instruments of Remote Sensing have relied on reflected solar radiation, but a fundamentally new kind of instrument, developed at the Jet Propulsion Laboratory of the California Instititute of Technology, in the U.S.A. was put into orbit aboard the NASA spacecraft Seasat in 1978. This instrument carried its own radar system to direct its radiation onto the Earth and synthesize an image from the reflected radiation.

Since an orbiting radar system provides its own 'illumination' it does not rely on the light of the Sun. It can therefore 'see' equally during day and night and can provide uninterrupted imaging of phenomena such as migrating ice floes. Radar frequencies, unlike ordinary light, penetrate cloud and fog and provide images in all kinds of weather and can photograph areas that are for long periods inaccessible to ordinary light. Further, since microwave frequencies used in radar penetrate the surface of the Earth to some depth, radar has provided information that is undetectable with instruments that rely on the Sun.

For example, a second radar system called SIR-A (Shuttle Imaging Radar-A) carried on board NASA space shuttle Columbia in 1981 revealed ancient river beds buried 1-3 metres below the surface in the Sahara Desert, and fossil drainage system in Egypt were identified at depths of up to 6 metres under the smooth desert sand. The same mission also gave first information about important geological features in heavily forested areas of Indonesia and Brazil.

Computers are the hub of Remote Sensing. The data collected by remote sensors is transmitted back to ground stations on Earth in digital form. Afterwards it is manipulated repeatedly in a variety of ways to analyze it, to turn it into images and patterns and to elicit information from masses of submerged clues that the human eye by itself is powerless to perceive .

Meterology, climatology and oceanography are the sciences that began to benefit immediately from Remote Sensing but such information is now being used on a widespread front in managing the health of the environment. Monitoring of vegetational changes for crop area estimation, yield prediction, stress and disease detection, motions of oil slicks and other kinds of pollutions, breeding grounds of locusts in desert areas, iceberg production and migration in fjords (these are hazards to shipping) are some examples of activities that have relied recently on Remote Sensing. One of the most significant actions of Remote Sensing has been to demonstrate the ability of radar carrying instruments to penetrate desert surfaces covered in very dry sand. This information is expected to be of very great value in understanding climatic change and managing resources in desert environments as discussed below.

Remote Sensing in understanding the ecology of arid lands

Unlike the advanced imaging tools of medicine described in the last section, whose benefits are at present directed almost entirely at the people living in rich countries, the benefits of Remote Sensing are being felt globally. We give below an example of its usage in the service of some of the poorest people in the world.

One of the severest environmental malaise is the spread of desert areas in many parts of the world. Pictures of mass starvation from arid lands in Africa in recent years have shown how devastating the consequences can be.

Whereas in the short term, emergency food and other supplies can mitigate the problem, long term solutions demand a scientific understanding of the ecology of these lands. Remote Sensing combined with other scientific methods is being used to further such understanding and also to offer practical advice of more immediate benefit.

For example, the Overseas Development Directorate of the Commission of the European Communities is funding the programme 'Programme Contre le Faim' - programme against hunger - in a number of African states. Among other applications, the programme is using Remote Sensing as an aid to agricultural management. Satellite tracking of rain clouds can provide a reliable method of recording rainfall over large areas. Satellite imagery, supported by ground observations, can also be used to map and monitor vegetation and to understand the relationship between observed rainfall, soils, vegetation growth and the intensity of use of the pastureland by grazing animals.

Meteorological satellites armed with Remote Sensing are making available valuable meteorological advice to farmers in arid lands allowing them to choose the right species and the right time and cultivate. Such advice is of crucial importance in these lands where not only the amount but the pattern of rainfall determines whether or not there is adequate yield to support the community.

Surprising though it may seem, drought-induced famine is not always due to the absence of rain. In Niger, for example, the total rainfall figures for 1984 recorded a normal year, yet the drought killed much of the harvest and led to widespread starvation. This anomaly arose because it rained only at the beginning and end of the rainy season. At the critical period in the middle, when the young crops needed water to survive and mature, there was none. In such climates, knowing the most opportune time for ploughing, planting and weeding can lead to a bumper crop but without this knowledge the outcome can be just a barren dust bowl.

Remote Sensing observations combined with other ecological information will also allow herds to be grazed productively and efficiently therby checking the advance of desert, a great deal of which has previously been induced through over-grazing.

The coupling of Remote Sensing, computer modelling and other ecological methods has already helped quite dramatically in some instances. Amid the recent devastation in Africa, a relative success story has been that of Botswana. By 1986 the country had suffered five consecutive years of drought, yet the people had managed to to avoid mass starvation. This was achieved through efficient management based on the forecasts of a computer model and the advice of meteorologists, agriculturists and agronomists.

The computer model has been developed by the UN's Food and Agriculture Organisation and is known as the Agrometeorological Crop Monitoring and Forecasting Model (AGROMET). The model is supplied with information on rainfall and evaporation rates. From this it calculates a factor called the "water stress" for various crops. This allows the computer to forecast crop yield in advance and so resources can be diverted to cope with possible emergencies.

The computer model once again emphasies the link between survival and information. Before AGROMET became available, officials had to rely on data gathered as the crops actually matured and the information took weeks to reach the offices from where actions to meet the effects of crop failures are directed.

Environmental Impact Analysis

The biggest worldwide concern regarding the environment is to prevent it being damaged, polluted and disfigured through the effects of human actions. The science of Environmental Impact Analysis has grown to cater for this concern. Its object is to predict the consequences of such things as new power plants, dams, motorways, forest plantations etc. on environmental factors such as plant and animal life, noise, drainage characteristics and so on. The visual impact of such activities also requires consideration. We may, for example, need to visualise how the pylons of a future power line will alter the scenic and aesthetic attributes of a site.

To make such predictions the computer utilises a mixture of analytical and portrayal techniques. Analysis involves such activities as data collection, statistical processing and modelling. Typically, the computer is being used to collect data and characterise the physical and biological atributes of all lakes and rivers in Britain. This information is being used to assess environmental impacts of various developments and to construct computer models for future predictions.

Portrayal techniques, on the other hand, are used to produce graphical images which can then be used for visualisation. Typically, SCOPE and PREVIEW are two programs used by the US Forest Service to visualise long-term consequences of tree harvesting and growth. In visual impact analysis, the trend is to combine computer images of planned future structures with actual photographs of a site. These result in computerised versions of photomontages and much research is currently in progress to improve methods of producing these.

Environmental information systems

There is virtually no limit to the types of environmental information that are needed - information about mountains, volcanoes, cities, airports, footpaths, motorways, plant life, mineral deposits, disease distributions, administrative boundaries, mortality rates and so on. All sorts of maps and tables have been constructed over the centuries to record and convey such information.

Naturally, the computer is increasingly active in handling and displaying environmental information. There are many forms of computerised systems for handling such information. The simple ones merely record information on one subject and facilitate its retreival, updating and presentation in terms of maps and tables. For example some plant and animal life recording systems used by botanists and zoologists do just that. Others offer greater automation. For example one microcomputer-based counting system has automated the recording of plankton (free-floating plants and animals in water).

Systems for the sharing of environmental information to improve administrative efficiency are now extensively being developed and used. For example, an information system called CORINE developed by the Institute of Terrestrial Ecology in UK is now being used by the administrators of the European Economic Community in Brussels to protect the European environment. CORNIE provides up-to-date information about the state of rivers, landscape and wildlife throughout the member states.

In many situations, the facility to combine information from many sources is a major requirement. The power of the computer really comes into play in meeting this requirement. We now look at an example.

An environmental information systems for school: The Domesday Project

A interesting environmental information which illustrates the power of the computer to combine data from a mutiplicity of observations has come from the recently completed Domesday Project, organised in the UK by the BBC. First we look briefly at the background.

The Norman king of England, William the Conquerer, instigated a fascinating and from the standards of the day a mammoth exercise in data collection and analysis in the Middle Ages. In the year 1086 his appointed agents conducted a through survey of England to collect detailed information about the land - how much?, what kind?, taxable value ?, about the people - whether freemen, servile or intermediate and about pigs, sheep and cows.

Somewhere between seven and nine circuits were designated, and commisioners appointed to make a county by county survey. The evidence was initially collected orally, and went through a series of courts and commissioners to finish up in the survey headquarters at Winchester. Finally, two volumes resulted; volume 1 giving a summary of observations and volume 2 giving detailed informations. These books now reside in the Public Records Office in London.

To celebrate the 900th aniversary of the original Domesday project the BBC organised a modern computer-based version of the same exercise which was completed in September 1986. Around 14000 schools and various other community groups such as ramblers, naturalists and others were alloted 4X3 kilometre blocks and asked to record their personal views of that area of their local environment familiar to them. This information was combined with photographs, TV and film images, satellite pictures from Remote Sensing, references and a vast array of statistical information .

The finished product became available in early 1987 on two LV-ROM (Laser Vision Read Only Memory) discs. One of the discs, the Community Disc, contains maps, diagrams, photographs and text as submitted by school children and other non-specialist data gatherers. The other one, called the National Disc, contains statistical information and contributions from professionals. On one of its sides there are 120 short TV/film clips of events, reported mainly in news and sport, in Britain. The other side contains specially commissioned photographs, selected essays and statistical information about life in Britain.

Not only has the computer made possible an amazing mine of environmental information on tap, but made it available in an extraordinarily friendly way. To use the system the user simply manipulates a mouse or a trackerball to move an onscreen pointer which selects from a set of options in a menu bar. Typically, by selecting the option PHOTOS, the user can go through a hierarchy of photographs - from satellite shots right down to local maps presented by school children. He can obtain pictures, diagrams, grid references, statistics and all sorts of other environmental information on castles, cathedrals, rivers, birds and so on. One interesting option on the National Disc offers the user nine different computer animated "walks" around an "Art Gallery" to examine statues, pictures and architectural details. There is much more and at all times there is a HELP option available to clarify the meaning of the displayed options. It's all a remarkably enjoyable way to discover environmental information and it shows how information will be presented increasingly in the future.

Computers in the analysis of complex environmental problems

It is estimated that through human actions, such as the burning of coal, the concentration of carbon dioxide in the Earth's atmosphere has increased by about 25 percent since the middle of the last century. This is causing the Earth to warm up. A set of four reports published by the U.S. Department of Energy in 1986 suggests that this effect - called the 'greenhouse effect' may increase temperatures to levels unattained for 100,000 years.

The above is just one of many examples of highly complex environmental problems which we seek to understand. It is recognised that through natural causes, such as the slowly changing tilt of the Earth's axis in its orbit around the sun, as well as through human intervention of the kind described above, our environment is constantly changing in ways that have profound implications for our future survival.

Only about 5000 years ago the Sahara desert was dotted with lakes and swamps and life could flourish there abundantly. Today it is parched and barren. How can we detect subtle changes that lead to catastrophic long-term effects and how can we respond to them wisely? How has the climate changed over the last million years? How much pollution can be tolerated without making unsafe our fish stocks? How long before the oil and coal reserves run out? How can we promote industrial development and maintain ecological balance? Will the ice age return? Is drinking-water connected with heart disease? - there are many such pressing questions to answer.

Computer analysis and modelling are the only tools we possess to attack such highly complex problems. We have to grant that despite the aid of the mightiest supercomputers, our answers to questions concerning the future of our environment and its resources at present remain frought with major uncertainties. For example, computer predictions of the greenhouse effect have been dismissed by some researchers as being entirely wrong whereas others such as Carl Sagan have defended them for twenty years.

The discrepancies between various forecasts of the future of the Earth's resources are equally wide. Not so long ago the last U.S. President Jimmy Carter commissioned a study called *Global 2000*. This predicted that by the end of century, resulting from large population increases, there would be mass depletion of the Earth's resources leading to widespread malnutrition and poverty. *The Resourceful Earth,* published only a few years later in 1984 during the presidency of Ronald Reagan states categorically that "Environmental resource and population stresses are diminishing and with the passage of time will have less influence than now upon the quality of human life on our planet".

Despite the shakiness of our current powers of prediction, we are obliged to indulge in the exercise. Choices that may have crucial consequences have to be made. Society has to plan and legislate. There are good theoretical reasons to suspect that many complex environmental processes are of the type where the long-term outcome cannot be predicted. In that case we have to seek the best partial, tentative and short-term information that we can discover.

Granted that we may never be able to predict the future very far ahead, there is no doubt that with increases in computer power, computer analysis and modelling will begin to offer insight into many complex situations that are currently shrouded in uncertainty. We now look at two examples of this kind.

Weather forecasting

Weather forecasting is very representative of the kind of complexity met with in modelling intricate environmental processes and we can gain insight into the possibilities by examining what has happened in this field.

Computer modelling of the weather has consistently improved as the storage capacities and the speed of computers have increased. For example, in 1959, the U.K. Meteorological Office installed its first computer which was able to perform 3000 arithmetical operations per second. Its present day supercomputer successor can perform 400 million of such operations in the same time.

Each major increase in computer power has made it possible to add further refinements to the computer programs used to model the weather, which has improved the accuracy of the forecast. For example, during the 1970s the accuracy of the 48-hour forecast improved to match the accuracy of the 24-hour one of a decade earlier. With the supercomputer, forecasts that display very fair accuracy are being made five days ahead and the ones for 72 hours ahead have attained very highly accuracy indeed.

In modelling phenomena such as the weather, billions of computations have to be performed and even with today's supercomputers the task becomes possible only through accepting crude approximations to real effects . For example, in the model employed by the U.K. Meteorological Office, the average values of temperature, pressure, humidity and wind speed are used for an area covering 150 square kilometers. Clearly, there can be a lot of variation in such a large area and the present resolution is far from ideal.

With further advancements in computer power and in methods of observation, computer models of similar environmental processes will continue to become more realistic and accurate. Although, as was said earlier, it is possible that there are fundamental principles at work, such as the effects of atmospheric turbulence in weather forecasting, which limit the timescales over which we can forecast environmental changes. It is also clear, however, that these limits are at present far from having been attained.

Epidemiology

In Tanzania, Uganda and Kenya three out of every 1000 children below the age of 15 are hit by a cancerous malignancy known as Burkitt's lymphoma which commonly affects the jaw, yet an area of about 200 square miles in the midst of the affected region is practically free from it.

In the North-West Normandy and Brittany regions of France the incidence of the cancer of the oesophagus is 18 times higher than in the rest of Europe.

The inhabitants of the North or West of England and Wales have a lower life expectancy than the inhabitants of South or East. The differences are quite large and increased mortality rates applicable over a wide range of diseases.

Such striking patterns of 'hot spots' and 'cold spots' in incidence of disease occur for many diseases all over the world. How can these be explained ? In the case of England and Wales, the weather, soft drinking water, smoking habits, consumption of fruit and vegetable, rates of unemployment have all been suggested as likely factors.

Clearly environmental and life style factors must be at work but to pin them down has not always been easy and many major epidemiological problems, though recorded over a considerable period, remain unsolved. Such is the case for the North-South divide found in England and Wales which has been known for one hundred years.

The lack of success in finding clear answers to such problems is easy to understand. The task of collecting, disentangling and correlating the data is laborious and highly unwieldy. If the same people who smoke heavily are also the people who suffer from bad housing, unemployment, lack of exercise, soft drinking water and broken homes then it is not easy to disentangle whether or not soft water is a significant factor in the incidence of heart disease. Here then is another example of an environmental problem containing many interacting factors which cannot be isolated and studied separately.

Computers, once again, constitute the only tool that offer some hope of providing scientific answers to such problems. For this reason, many computer-based studies on a global scale under the aegis of the United Nations World Health Organisation, as well as many national studies are in progress to try to identify the causes of environmental factors in disease. These involve massive amounts of data collection and statistical analysis.

For example, the USA is aiming to reduce the incidence of cancer by half within the next fifteen years and the National Cancer Institute in Washington DC is currently conducting 26 computer-aided prevention trials to examine the effects of diet, smoking and exposure to carcinogens in the environment.

The Japanese have also been highly active in epidemiological studies and one of their recent contributions concerns the value of eating green vegetables everyday. For example, a 16-year study on 122261 men carried out by the National Cancer Research Institute in Tokyo showed that those who did not smoke or drink, did not eat meat every day but did eat a daily helping of green vegetables, ran one-fifth the the risk of developing cancer of the mouth, pharynx, oesophagus and lungs, and half the risk of developing heart disease, peptic ulcers and other cancers. A similar study on 26518 men and women showed that non-smoking wives of smoking husbands also carried a higher risk of heart disease and cancer but again, a daily helping of green vegetables reduced the risk incurred from cigarette smoke in the environment.

A major success of epidemiology in recent years has been the certain identification of cigarette smoking as the environmental trigger in most lung cancers. Such single clear cut answers are, however, only rarely to be found. Nevertheless, thanks to computer power, the studies now in progress will undoubtedly help to disentangle some of the myths from facts and put preventive advice and legislation on a more scientific footing.

Computers and Sport

Sport is a reflection of society. As society's values and methods change, so do those of sport. Since the computer is now the prime tool of the technically developed society we would expect it to be prominent in sport and so indeed it is.

Whereas until about the mid-1960s innate talent and 'amateurism' could lead to the heights in competitive sport, it is now becoming more and more necessary to seek a partnership with science and technology. The training of today's champions demands a sophisticated understanding of such things as the physiology and anatomy of limbs, the function of heart and lungs, the biochemistry of muscle action, the psychology of the 'resolve to win' and the ergonomic design of equipment. Not surprisingly, at the very pinnacle of sport 'move over coach - here come the computers' is beginning to be the trend.

Of course, at the levels where sport is more for fun and enjoyment, rather than for fierce gladiatorial combat, the situation is rather different. Nevertheless, computers are beginning to play a variety of roles even at the club and the individual level. Just as the materials that were originally developed for space vehicles have found their way into non-stick kitchen utensils, so some of the computerised aids being developed for champions will be passed down to serve the ordinary individual. In this section we shall examine some of the key uses of computers in sport.

Biomechanics

We saw in the two earlier sections that the computer made a fundamental impact in medicine and environmental sciences through making available powerful new tools of observation. The same kind of impact has also occured in top-level sport.

In any sport there are two problems facing the participant. Firstly, to produce and sustain an optimum level of effort for some period and secondly to channel this energy efficiently into the desired task - rather than frittering it away in wasteful action or sustaining injury. Biomechanics is concerned with improving the efficiency of action so as to be able to extract the best possible performance.

The basic ideas of biomechanics are easy to grasp. Suppose that a javelin thrower can generate a certain maximum amount of power. His throw will depend not only on this power but also on the efficiency with which energy is concentrated in the throwing arm and then transferred to the javelin. The angle at which the javelin is released is another key factor. The same principles of mechanics that are used to predict the orbit of a space satellite can be used to predict what will happen to the javelin if we can find out the forces applied to it by the thrower's body. From basic anatomical information about the weights of different segments of the body and from detailed observations of the motions of the performer the information about the forces can be calculated mathematically using laws which have been known for three hundred years, since Sir Isaac Newton observed the fall of his apple.

Biomechanics combines high speed photography and computers to obtain this information. It is being used to give scientific insights into why the great champions win and to suggest to others how they could emulate them.

Although the principles behind biomechanics have been known for more than two hundred years, their application in top level sport was pioneered by Dr. Gideon Ariel as recently as the early 1970s. He is a former Israeli athlete who competed in the discus in the 1960 and 1964 Olympics and who in now a major consultant in the coaching of elite athletes in America. His company, Computerised Biomechanical Analysis, formed in 1971, was the first to make this kind of analysis available commercially.

In Ariel's analysis, a high speed cine film is first produced of the athlete in action - anything from 64 to 10000 frames. The film is then projected frame by frame onto a digisiter screen. By directing a special pen-like device onto such a screen the position of any point touched by the pen is transmitted for storage and processing by a computer. The positions of the crucial joints in the body such as the shoulders, knees and ankles are digitised from the cine frames. This information, together with anatomical information on the athlete's body, is processed by the computer to calculate the forces generated during the action. By joining the points digitised, the computer also produces a graphic display of moving 'stick figures' which show the essentials needed for diagnostics and coaching.

The actions performed by various segments of the body such as the arms, feet, ankles and so on can then be analysed and compared with the actions of champions. The computer can also show how changes in the positioning and movements of the various segments of the body will affect performance. Very often minute changes can lead to substantial gains.

Ariel's work first hit the headlines about a decade ago. He analysed the action of of the American discus thrower Mac Wilkins and discovered that Wilkins' front leg

70

was wastefully absorbing energy that could be channeled into his throwing. This analysis led Wilkins to modify his technique. He increased his performance by about 4 metres and went on to win the gold medal in the 1976 Olympics.

Since Wilkins' win, Ariel's coaching has chalked up impressive successes with many other sportsmen and sportswomen. A world record by Terry Albritton in the shot put and an addition of 10 mph to Jimmy Connors' already formidable 70 mph tennis service, victories for the US Olympic Women's Volleyball team are just a few examples of triumphs that have come through minor but crucial changes in technique. Because it offers insight not only about the performer but also about the performer's rivals, computerised biomechanics can be doubly effective. Ariel has used it, for example, to analyse the Bulgarian, Soviet and East German gold medal winning weight lifters.

Another computer-based diagnostic tool of biomechanical analysis is the force platform. This is a highly sensitive electronically wired platform for measuring the intensity and direction of applied body forces. It is being used by cyclists, for example, to measure the forces applied to the pedals and so tell whether both legs are working equally effectively. Archers, on the other hand, use the platform to detect the minutest sway in their stance (only about a millimetre can divert the arrow by 10 centimetres by the time it reaches the target). The US Olympic Committee has set up the so called Elite Athletes Programme with 15 research centres to offer scientific training methods to top athletes from more than a dozen sports and the force platform is one of the key tools on offer.

Although biomechanics has mostly been publicised as the technique for the coaching of Olympic champions, this in fact is a very narrow area of its application. Not only world-class performers but most individuals are interested in improving performance to a satisfying level and learning to identify their personal idiosyncracies. Biomechanics can be usefully employed in coaching at every level and indeed it has been so used at many colleges and universities for many years. In the U.K., for example, Dr. Mike Lindsay of Leeds University has worked extensively with it and has developed a 3-D system employing three cameras. With the growing power of microcomputers there is no doubt that biomechanical analysis will become very widely available for coaching in all major sporting activities.

Sporting activities are of course not the only kind of activities that demand efficient use of the body. Indeed everyone needs to learn good body use and we shall have more to say on this in the next chapter. The two other major areas where good body use can be crucial in avoidance of pain and injury have to do with disability and occupational stress.

Biomechanical analysis is therefore fundamental in designing aids to cope with physical handicaps and occupational strains. For example, to ease the backache of a surgeon from his prolonged stooping over an operating table, biomechanical analysis led to the design of a special harness and modifications to his shoes. A well-known company has utilised biomechanical analysis to design an elasticated nappy for infants with defective knee and hip joints.

At the University of Waterloo in Canada a computerised 'Gait Laboratory' has been set up to study muscle interaction in order to find out how surgery and physiotherapy can help the disabled to walk more comfortably. The laboratory is also investigating the deterioration of muscles with ageing and among other topics, they are studying how and why we lose the spring in our step as we grow older. One of their findings that deserves to be more widely known is that most joggers are misguided about how to exercise their legs; whereas most try to concentrate on developing the thigh muscles, the emphasis should be on the calf muscles which sustain forces from three to eight times greater.

Computers in the evaluation of personal characteristics of champions

Since the 1920s it has been increasingly appreciated that the ability to determine the most suitable physique and constitution for each kind of event in athletics is as important for top level performance as the training methods. The pioneering study on the subject was carried out in Germany by W. Kohlraush who analysed body measurements of the participants in the Deutsche Kamfspiele held in Berlin in 1925 and of those who competed in the 9th Olymics held in 1928 in Amsterdam. He concluded that performers fell into recognisable groups and described the characteristics of sprinters, middle and long distance runners, and others such as swimmers and throwers. Since then many more studies have been carried out and a very detailed understanding has been built up not only of the physique required but also of other physiological factors that make for success in various fields.

For example, as far as physique is concerned, a top class high jumper must ideally be tall and have long legs relative to the trunk so as to possess a high centre of gravity. His muscles require the qualities of elasticity and spring rather than great explosive power as in the case of a shot putter's arm. Muscle has been classified into different types of fibre, each with its own characteristic type of contraction. Individuals have their own, genetically detetermined fibre mix. A person with a higher proportion of so called slow twitching muscle fibres to the fast twitching ones is suited to endurance events rather than those requiring short bursts of explosive action, and so on.

Thus, apart from advanced training methods, top sports competitors need expert evaluation of their individual physiologies and other personal characteristics. 'Know thyself' is the key injunction for anyone who aims to go far.

We have already seen that biomechanics provides highly detailed information about an individual's physical actions. Computers are also involved in providing similar information on a whole range of personal characteristics, e.g. on bodytype, body fat and many other physiological measurements. In the Elite Athlete

Programme of the US Olympics Committee, for example, computer analysis provides a highly detailed physiological profile of each athlete which is recorded over a long period. For any particular performer, the training programme, the diet, the optimum target body weight etc. all take account of this personal profile.

Keeping a record of performance in training is also vital. The paperwork involved in recording information without the use of a computer is highly tedious. By eliminating form filling, the computer makes it much easier to record details of training and progress. Another requirement is to be able to compare one's own progress with that of one's past and present peer competitors. Whereas this is easy with a computer, it is highly time-consuming otherwise. The computer can keep up-to-date information about performances of others, national and international averages and so on and analyse and display progress effortlessly. It can suggest an optimum path to peak performance for a scheduled event. These facilities also make for effective coaching. The coach can keep a detailed eye on the trainee without having to be physically present in the same place.

Sports injuries

Top sportsmen and women of today are stressed to extremes and much scientific work is being done in sports medicine to learn about the avoidance of injury. Great advances have occured in the last decade in the understanding of muscle physiology and have lead to accelerated methods of rehabilitation. However, the subject depends on more than just a knowledge of muscle physiology.

Intrinsic to the avoidance of injuries is the understanding and correction of injury patterns. It has been observed that the same kinds of injuries recur repeatedly to individuals as well as to groups. Apart from developing better methods of treatment, another challenge lies in being able to predict the circumstances under which a certain type of injury is most likely to occur and to take preventive measures in advance. It is also necessary to teach sportsmen and women to learn to manage their bodies on sound physiological principles.

We have already seen that computers are active in helping to improve technique. They are also helping to reduce injuries. For example, at Pennsylvania State University, the National Athletic Injuries Reporting Sytem (NAIRS) has used computers since the mid-1970s in helping to identify and reduce patterns of injury. NAIRS covers the whole range of sport - swimming, diving, athletics, basketball, American Football and so on.

The computer processes several hundred highly detailed reports each week from a multitude of sporting institutions such as colleges, universities and clubs. Apart from the personal details of the injured party, the diagnosis and the type and duration of treatment, these carry detailed information about injuries sustained. Information such as whereabouts on the playing field; the type of playing surface; a description of the equipment and the kit; is recorded. The injuries are classified into 'minor' or 'significant', the minor ones being those which prevent participation for no more than a day.

The analysis is valuable for several reasons. Firstly, the computer alerts the sporting community to the introduction of something dangerous. Some new form of kit, training method or fashion may introduce a new pattern of injury. Secondly, the analysis provides quantitative information about risk factors associated with participation in different sports. We cannot give scientific answers to questions such as 'should middle-aged men play squash?' unless we have data available to support our assertions. The computer can tell us more accurately what is dangerous and what is not. Finally, the analysis is highly valuable to administrators. First aid and other medical services have to be provided for sporting events. The guidance on the level at which provision should be made for an event and its location and concentration on the field is provided by the computer.

The need for guidance on prevention of injury is clearly widespread and the micro can make a valuable contribution in the gym as well as at home. One of the major gaps in today's gymnasia is the absence of easy 'help' facilities to teach people about proper use of such items as the weight training equipment. The charts provided on walls are barely adequate for this purpose and injuries are quite common. Dynamic display is needed to convey full information and increased use of computer graphics, possibly in combination with interactive video, should make it easy to provide these. Education in emergency first aid will also benefit from such provisions.

Other uses

We have now considered some of the major ways in which the computer is being used in the service of sport. There remain many other possibly less glamourous but nevertheless vital roles. Organisation of sporting activities, mangement of facilities, selections of players and umpires, preparation of ranking order are typical examples. One rapidly developing application has to do with the analysis of tactics. The idea is to glean tactical information from the analysis of data from previous events, exactly as the chess masters remember the great historic moves that have led to victory. For example, in the U.K., computers are being used at Jordanhill College of Education in Glasgow and at Leeds Polytechnic to analyse badminton strategy and at Liverpool Polytechnic for strategy in hockey. The Football Association, the organising body for soccer in U.K, has supported this kind of research for its interest and similar programs are being developed for all team games.

It will be unfair to end this section without paying a tribute to the computer in enhancing of the enjoyment of sport for millions. When the Olympic games were held in Los Angeles in 1932 there was no such thing as TV and only a few thousand could watch them live. When the last Olympics returned there in 1984 TV pictures were beamed to more than two billion people around the world and half the world's population could follow the action. Behind the scenes the computer manages all sorts of operations to make the viewing enjoyable.

The instant display of information on times, distances, records, as well as the provision of other interesting information for commentators and observers is all handled by the computer. Then there is the editing of the picture for special effects. For this the TV picture is digitised and stored in computer memory. It can then be processed to change the size, contrast, perspective, colour and so on and played at various speeds. Without all this the picture on the flat screen would not be a very exciting prospect.

Finally, the author is at a loss to decide whether computer dating is medicine, ecology or sport. If it is one of these then it is appropriate to say that the computer is active in helping humans to do it.

References & Suggestions for Further Reading

1. B. Kostrewski (Editor), "Current Perspectives in Health Computing", Cambridge University Press, 1984. *This book is for the profesional medic who wants to obtain a good overview of the application of information technology in medicine. It charts the application of computers in health care in U.K. but is representative of what is happening in most of the other advanced countries.*
2. Pykett, I. L., "NMR Imaging in Medicine", Scientific American, May 1982. *Of all the imaging tools described in this book, probably NMR is potentially the most promising in medicine as well as sport. This article can be consulted for more information on the principles of NMR.*
3. "Molecules of life", Scientific American, Oct 1985. *A very inspiring collection of articles from leading scientists in micro-biology. Contains many beautiful images from computer modelling. Suitable for the non-specialist reader.*
4. Elachi, C., "Radar Images of the Earth from Space", Scientific American, December 1982. *Remote sensing using radar beams is the latest technique for observing the environment. This article is from a research scientist at the Jet Propulsion Laboratory who pioneered the method.*
5. Saunders, P., "Micros for Handicapped Users", Helena Press. 1985. *Contains a list of useful addresses and contacts. Also, in U.K., the BBC have produced a very useful little booklet entitled "With a Little Help From the Chip" which contains a fund of useful information. The booklet was produced to back up a TV series of the same name which ran in early 1986.*

6. New Scientist, 2 August 1984. *A good collection of articles for the general reader that show the role of science, technology and computers in top level sport.*
7. Brodie, D, and Thornhill, J., "Microcomputing in Sport and Physical Education", Lepus Books, 1983. *An excellent book that shows how the microcomputer is being used in this field. Contains many programs and would be of interest to all teachers of Physical Education.*

4. Computers in Personal Programmes of Fitness

The previous chapter looked at the way the computer is being used through organised social effort in medicine, environmental sciences and sport. Our purpose now is to show how the computer can help the individual to construct a personalised programme for the promotion of health and self preservation in a more autonomous way.

It is a fact that whereas methods of organised scientific medicine and competitive sports have made enormous strides in recent decades, the health culture (by which we shall mean the things that people do themselves to look after their own wellbeing rather than things that are done by experts when they are unwell - the latter should more accurately be referred to as the 'disease culture') remains astonishingly naive and fragmented. It bristles with contradictions, confusions and fads. It over-emphasises secondary features but fails to cater for the deeper needs.

"Teach him to live rather than to avoid death: life is not breath but action, the use of our senses, mind, faculties, every part of ourselves which makes us conscious of our being", so implored Jean-Jacques Rousseau two hundred years ago.

Despite such exhortations over the centuries, there is a conspicuous absence of any courses on *living,* developing the senses, mind, faculties etc. in any systematic and scientific way. Such instruction has remained random and perfunctory.

Although, science and technology have indeed invaded the gymnasia, their thrust has so far remained focussed on a very limited front. One only has to note the ancient origins of words such as 'Yoga', 'marathon' etc. and recipes such as a 'vegetarian diet' to recognise that what is on offer in mass culture mostly comprises repackaged goods that have been around for thousands of years.

Only a moment's reflection is needed to be able to grasp that mere variations on running, lifting, jumping, dancing and eating cannot possibly exercise all the grey matter that humans possess. After all even an average greyhound can outrun an Olympic sprinter and even a very mediocre kangaroo can outjump any star jumper, despite the equipment they clearly lack in their skull.

Granted that a well-balanced diet and the exercise of our muscles, heart and lungs is absolutely crucial, there clearly remains much else to *exercise* which profoundly determines our health.

For example, the great choreographer Blanchine was once asked when he was in his eighties, "how is it that you grow more youthful and vigorous with age?' He replied, "I have more energy now than when I was in my youth because I now know exactly what I want to do. It is confusion and lack of clarity in purpose that exhaust people, whatever their age".

Research has amply confirmed that lack of clarity in purpose is indeed a major cause of stress. For example, in November 1976 the National Association of Schoolmasters and the Union of Women Teachers in U.K. published a report on the growing stress in the teaching profession. The report revealed that deaths among male teachers had more than doubled compared to the decade previous and that the number qualifying for a breakdown pension had more than trebled. Anxious teachers suffered headaches, stomach upsets, body rashes, insomnia, hypertension and a whole variety of depressive illnesses causing some to end up "as emotionally drained husks".

The report pin-pointed the major cause of this condition as "role conflict and role ambiguity ".

Other research in cardio-vascular disease, the major killer in the developed world, has similarly highlighted lack of clarity in the occupational environment as a major culprit. Yet compared to the publicity given to smoking and cholesterol as risk factors, little has been done to highlight this factor. A survey conducted throughout USA by Dr. Robert Kahn of the University of Michigan Institute for Social Research found that 35 percent of the sample questioned suffered from lack of clarity in purpose and responsibilities, yet literature and advice on health in USA and elsewhere remains obsessed only with such things as pedalling bicycles and the eternal search for ever more healthful diets.

The above is just one example chosen to make the point that humans do not live by pumping biceps and watching waist lines alone. Given the rudiments of survival and freedom from genetic and other accidental misfortunes, health springs most essentially from the feeling of self esteem. Our self esteem is in turn dependent on our imagination and on our *effectiveness* in our environment. Thus an exercise system for humans must systematically promote the development of a positive imagination and of behaviour patterns that maximise the effectiveness of an individual in his environments.

The kind of health skills that need to be developed by persons living and competing in a technically advanced environment are self knowledge, efficient management of time, capacity to absorb information rapidly, capacity to get things done, self discipline, clear goals, good memory, good powers of communication with others, capacity for relaxation in the face of stress and change, and so on. A regime that merely promotes the ability to touch the toes can hardly qualify as a great health builder, yet this is the level at which 'look good', 'feel good' health recipes are currently promoted.

This crude sub-human approach may have been reasonably adequate when life expectancy was exceedingly low but it is now in need of drastic upgrading. The extension of the muscle-centred workout becomes crucial as middle age begins to set in, when the brain becomes subject to deterioration. Recent accurate measurements of brain volume have shown that the rate at which individuals lose irreplaceable brain cells is correlated with the quality of intellectual demand in their occupation. Professor Taiju Matsuzawa and colleagues at Tohoku National University in Japan measured brain volumes of a thousand people of different ages and professions. They observed significant cell loss in some subjects who were still in their thirties, yet in some who were in their seventies there was no evidence of deterioration.

When they examined the occupations of their subjects they found that farm workers, shop assistants and others doing routine jobs had lost cells more rapidly compared to lawyers and university professors.

It has also been demonstrated in laboratory experiments that mental activities of various kinds increase cerebral blood flow and hence the flow of oxygen and other nutrients to the brain cells. It is therefore reasonable to expect that sclerosis (the hardening of the brain arteries), which happens to be one of the major causes of senility and premature ageing, can be significantly reduced through a shift from a cardio-vascular to a cerebro-vascular health culture. Since life expectancy has steadily grown and since there are now growing ageing populations in every country this shift is urgently needed. This is undoubtedly the best recipe for the elixir of youth that humans presently possess.

One major reason why the health culture has remained frozen in a rudimentary state has had to do with the non-availability of an appropriate tool. Humans differ so much in their minds, faculties etc. that unless one is to turn out uniform automata, one needs a tool that is infinitely adaptable. Yet another reason is that factors such as smoking and cholestrol are, for the expert, easy and straightforward to identify and demand no great expenditure of their time. The experts neither have the time nor the skill to diagnose or promote such concepts as clarity of purpose. To promote such skills we need a tool that the individual can adapt and manipulate for himself.

For the first time in history we do possess such a tool in the computer. The exciting thing about the computer is not just that it can bring science to bear, vastly improving the traditional muscle-centred workout but that it can extend it to include non-motor functioning. The computer can interact with the whole spectrum of sensory and symbolic activity that a human brain is capable of producing. It can exercise the motor brain, the sensory brain, the emotional brain, the intellectual brain and the memory storing brain, all in an integrated way.

With well designed software, the computer can be readily adapted to cater for individual abilities, peculiarities and tastes. It can provide variety, novelty and surprise. It can free humans from the ancient hold of charismatic gurus and allow them to take charge of their own lives, which is undoubtedly the greatest health skill of all. It can, with proper research and development, lift the gymnasium out of the age of cavemen where it still resides and make it fit for humans living in the space age.

The purpose of this chapter is to show how computerised equipment can achieve all this to offer a more sophisticated approach to personal health and preservation. We first look at ways of improving the traditional muscle-centred activity. We then suggest some examples of extensions to cater for non-motor needs.

Computerised equipment for a personalised and systematic muscle-centred work out

There are more than 400 skeletal muscles in the body. An ideal exercise routine would contract and stretch all the muscles efficiently. It would move all the joints through their full ranges. It would condition the cardio-respiratory system. The programme would take account of the individuals personal data, sex, age, somatotype (thin, fat or muscular build), level of fitness, peculiarities - e.g. excessive curvature of the spine, other constraints - e.g. can only spare 20 minutes on Tuesday evenings etc. The programme would monitor progress, set targets, coax the individual to improve and would record and display performance. The programme would be enjoyable and would suitably inject elements of novelty and surprise.

At present the average person does things haphazardly and inefficiently. Only the occasional lip service is paid to personal data and in group activity the programmes usually reflect what suits the guru rather than the participant. There is very little understanding of the need of novelty, and most people tend to repeat the same old thing over and over again.

The computer can be utilised to construct scientifically balanced programmes and to record personal data. One clear difference between the attitude of a champion and that of a mediocre individual is that the champion trains systematically, has clearly defined targets and records data. Although not all of us are going to aspire to become champions, nevertheless, because of the complexity of the musculo-skeletal system it is not possible to cater efficiently for all our needs without making use of science. Far more can be achieved in far less time if we use a scientific basis to design our training.

Equally important is the act of recording data. Science only becomes possible through the gathering of data. The great contribution made by Dr. Kenneth Cooper who sparked off aerobics was not that he found out that jogging is good for us. That had been suggested frequently from time immemorial. He found out how much jogging is good for us, and what should be our targets. He was able to achieve this through gathering data.

Without the use of a computer, the recording of personal information is time consuming and tedious, but with a well designed interactive computer program it need take a very small amount of extra effort.

If the computer is utilised in no other way than for the purposes of producing well-balanced programmes for muscle tone, joint mobility and aerobic fitness, together with recording of personal data, then these alone can make a major advance on the haphazard approaches of today.

Computerised equipment suitable for clubs, gymnasia and for personal use is now increasingly appearing on the market. For example, a computerised weight training machine known as Modar (Motor Driven Accomodating Resistance Machine) has recently been marketed in West Germany to improve on the kind in common use today. The user supplies personal data to a controlling computer on a floppy disc. The computer controls a special exercising arm which affords the correct variable resistence to match the load with muscle performance, giving benefit through a whole range of movement. In this way, the user gets a comprehensive work-out in less than half the time it takes using the traditional equipment. Modar is more efficient, safer and gives a printout of performance in each session if desired. This provides valuable insight into the quality of and progress during the workout.

In the USA, Dr. Gideon Ariel, whose work on biomechanics was described in the last chapter has produced sophisticated computerised weight training machines which he calls CES (computerised exercise system). These machines are designed to offer highly customised personal exercise programs and put resistive weight training into a new realm of possibilities for scientific application in health care, fitness and rehabilitation. They have the ability to run pre-programmed sequences of exercises as well as tailored individual sequences.

CES offers isotonic, isokinetic, isometric or combinations of these modes of exercise. It can monitor, control and modify the speed and the resistance of an exercise throughout its range of motion. It provides extensive and accurate measurements of movement and strength. It allows for storage and subsequent comparison and analysis of the individual's performance. The equipment is interactive, providing immediate audio and visual feedback information during exercise. The interface is user-friendly making it possible for anyone to learn to use the equipment easily which is a far cry from from what has been on offer so far. CESs have been promoted as 'Intelligent Systems for Rehabilitation and Fitness' and their many features certainly qualify them for the accolade.

MODAR and CES are examples of highly sophisticated computerised exercise equipment which the average individual would not be able to afford or have room for. Computerised equipment in the form of exercise bicycles, rowing machines and jogging machines, all suitable for home use, has also become available. Such equipment can also allow for a wide range of adjustment. For instance, the Aerobicycle marketed by Universal offers a wide variability of pedal settings. It can simulate such situations as a long steady uphill gradient, a rolling hilly terrain and so on. It can be set for pulse training requiring the maintenance of a constant pedal rate and it gives information about the number of calories being consumed with any exercise.

Micro-based expert systems which offer advice on exercise and lifestyle have also appeared, though they have so far failed to make any significant impact. There can be little doubt, however, that such systems will be used more extensively with advances in artificial intelligence and with improvements in the user interface possibly even including speech recognition.

Computers for the teaching of good body use

In the last chapter we explained how biomechanics has helped many champions to improve performance through teaching them how to use their bodies more effectively. A much cheaper and less sophisticated version of similar equipment could be exploited to rectify a major failing in today's health education.

The crucial significance of good 'posture', or more accurately, 'good dynamic body use', for the maintenance of health, avoidance of stress and preservation of youthfulness has been recognised and written about extensively. Indeed one highly respected medical scientist and author has gone so far as to suggest that 'the basic structure of the personality, at its minutest level, is fashioned from good BODY-USE' (see page 19, The Alexander Principle, by Dr. Wilfred Barlow, published by Gollancz). However, due to under-developed awareness in most individuals of the variations in movements of their body segments, the subject is very time-consuming to teach in a scientific way. Only physiotherapists, dancers, gymnasts and similarly trained persons possess a sufficiently developed awareness of their body movements to be able to appreciate the subtleties involved. For this reason, bad backs, slumped spines, flat feet, protruding bellies and grossly distorted necks continue to abound, leading to unnecessary suffering and premature ageing and stiffening. The misuse of the body results in enormous loss of productivity and provides rich pickings for the practioners of fringe medicine and quack science.

The stick figures of biomechanics, by eliminating the inessential and focussing on the movements of the key joints, convey information in a way that can be grasped with precision. Biomechanics, it has been demonstrated, can be employed to detect fraudulent health insurance claims for back injury. A genuine sufferer with incapacitating backache typically reports pain at the same body angle with only a 1% variation. Someone who is pretending cannot maintain the kind of accuracy that is measured by the equipment and so is exposed. The same techniques could be used effectively to give individuals an accurate awareness of how to deploy their backs, necks, pelvises etc. most effectively for the promotion of their health and fitness and the avoidance of stress.

Computers for the exercise of the sensory apparatus

In the forest, survival depends on the sharpness of the sensory apparatus. A creature must spot the food, the mate or a safe site for a nest before a competitor does the same. Being able to tell the difference between a safe bush and a cunningly camouflaged enemy is literally a matter of life and death.

Not surprisingly, more than eighty percent of brain matter is estimated to be involved in the processing of sensory information. The exercise of the sensory apparatus should therefore be regarded as essential in a programme of fitness.

With the availability of the computer there is no reason why a modern gym should ignore this fundamental need. Through the addition of suitable computerised equipment the usual exercise apparatus can be extended to cater for the senses. Such equipment should monitor the acuity of the senses and provide precise information about changes. It should exercise the various sensory components efficiently and systematically and push their functioning nearer towards their potential. It should provide much needed educational information about the workings and the care of the sensory apparatus. The exercise of the senses can equip the individual to celebrate the multitude of happenings in the environment that are sources of pleasure and wonderment to the possessor of acutely functioning senses.

We shall first select the sense of hearing, which happens to be a neglected and often abused sense in the urban environment, to illustrate what needs to be done and why. No highly specialised or expensive equipment would be needed in this case and the effort would pay great dividends. Later we shall comment on the needs of the other senses.

Hearing

Let us begin by reviewing some basic information on sound and hearing.

Sound is produced as a result of changes in air pressure caused by vibrating objects. These pressure changes are converted into electrical nerve impulses by the ear and transmitted to the brain for interpretation. The slightly different times of arrival of a sound at the left and the right ear are utilised by the brain to identify the location of a source of sound.

A sound is characterised by its intensity and frequency. The intensity of sound is measured in units of decibels. This is a logarithmic unit (goes up by powers of 10; a 10 decibel sound is twice as loud as a 1 decibel sound, but a 100 decibel sound is a thousand times louder). A very low intensity sound such as that produced by rustling leaves is of the order of 10 decibels, an ordinary conversation about 50 decibels, whereas a very loud pneumatic drill gives out something like a 100 decibels. Above about 115 decibels sound becomes painful and injurious.

It's worth remarking that the decibel is not a very suitable unit to convey the amazing range of perception of the human ear. The energy carried by the loudest sound that the ear can tolerate is a hundred thousand million times more than that carried by the faintest sound it can detect, which is about 10^{-14} Watts. If, by comparison, the eyes were as sensitive as the ears then an ordinary 60W bulb lit in London would be visible at distances comparable with those of New York, Ottawa and Baghdad !

Studies over the past twenty years or so have shown that exposure to noise and ageing both result in hearing loss at higher frequencies which normally stretch from 20 to 20,000 cycles per second. At least in the urban environment, it is unusual for persons aged over forty to be able to hear significantly above 10,000 cycles per second. Typically an average loss of about 30 decibels at higher frequencies for men in their 60's has been found to occur.

The extent to which hearing potential remains under-utilised and capable of development is perhaps best indicated by the achievements of blind persons. Many such persons not only overcome their handicap to cope well with the normal demands of living but have been known to become highly accomplished horsemen, swimmers, skiers and so on. These apparently superhuman accomplishments are achieved through the development of hearing to a level nearer its potential.

Erasmus Darwin, grandfather of Charles Darwin, described how his blind friend Justice Fielding on first visiting his room deduced accurately that the room was 22 feet long, 18 feet wide and 12 feet high. This is a classical description of the phenomena known as 'facial vision'. Sound waves bounce off surfaces and echo differently in different rooms, depending on the size, the numbers of open and shut doors, windows and so on. Persons who develop facial vision are able to interpret this 'ambience' with great accuracy. (A recent book that gives some vivid descriptions of this is authored by the blind Indian writer Ved Mehta - *The Ledge Between the Streams,* Harvill Press.)

Although it is generally assumed that deterioration in hearing is a normal and unavoidable consequence of the ageing process, there are findings which suggest that this view is erroneous and unduly pessimistic. Studies of some African tribes who live in quiet environments on the borders of the Sudan have, for example, discovered that the elder tribesmen show no loss in hearing at all. It would seem therefore that with proper care and exercise there is far greater potential, not only for development but also for preservation with age. Science ought to be able to do significantly better than what is achieved in complete ignorance.

The major reason for the unquestioning acceptance of deterioration is that the muscle-centred health culture fails to offer any programme for the care of the sensory apparatus. More than one million workers in Britain alone spend their working days in surroundings that damage their hearing. It has been known for some time that long-term deafness is a major cause of mental illness in the elderly. Yet of

84

the thousand and one books on jogging and dieting published each year, how many say anything about the care of the hearing apparatus?

Animals in the forest do not go jogging or weight lifting. They run in response to sensory stimuli - to find food, mate, shelter and so on. Problem solving and sensing activities occur simultaneously with the working of the cardio-vascular system. If we take a healthy dog for a walk, the dog does not just plod along jogging. It sniffs, scratches, goes after a cat, has a quarrel with another dog and so on. It instinctively gives its sensory apparatus a workout simultaneously with the motor workout.

If we think from an evolutionary perspective then it becomes very easy to predict that the best exercises would be those that would significantly couple motor and sensory activity. The reason why the oriental martial arts training produces so many remarkably agile old masters is that the exercises have a high sensory content.

Although evolutionary explanations have not been offered, many have empirically hit upon the benefits to be had from the addition of sensory activity to muscle-based exercise. Such was the case of the great Swedish athletics coach Gosta Olander. A keen naturalist and photographer of wild life, Olander was led through observations of wild animals to devise his training method which involved awareness training. This involved acute observations of the environment while out jogging. In the 1960s he trained dozens of world beating champion athletes and also brought physical fitness to thousands of ordinary people.

Computerised exercises for hearing

The scientific method for the design of exercise should firstly be based on an evolutionary perspective. We should begin by asking the question - what attributes have favoured the chances of survival over the evolutionary span? If we ask this about hearing, we conclude that survival has demanded five key hearing attributes. These are, the facilities to (i) hear a range of frequencies, (ii) recognise a range of sounds made by other creatures and objects in the environment, (iii) recognise the location of sources of sounds in the environment, (iv) select, focus and maintain attention on a source of sound (also blot out sounds that are not of interest) and (v) respond rapidly with appropriate motor actions to a particular sound.

To optimise our programmes we should design equipment and training methods that make demands on all these usages with increasing efficiency.

The facility to hear a range of frequencies at some minimal intensities is the primary attribute of good hearing. The value of computerised equipment to exercise hearing is easy to grasp. Such equipment would easily set and display the relevant intensities and frequencies. It would also perform a number of other useful functions. For example the computer would be able to set the intensity norm (i.e. what the average person of good hearing should be able to hear) automatically for a given frequency.

(1) In the basic exercise the user would simply listen with focussed attention to a set of sounds at discrete frequencies. These frequencies would sample the whole spectrum detectable to a normal human ear. Initially, the computer would set the intensity level at the norm and the user would gradually alter the setting, moving up or down, until the sound became just detectable.

(2) Another basic exercise would involve the matching of frequencies. In this, the computer would play a note at random. Then the subject, by twiddling a knob, would try to produce a matching sound. When the subject was convinced that the sound emanating was of the same frequency as that given out initially by the computer then some key would be pressed. The computer will then display information about the accuracy of the choice made. To relax the demand on short-term memory the facility to ask the computer to replay the sound could be made available.

(3) Exercises for recognising sounds can be built up quite easily and can cater for a wide range of tastes. For example, a popular TV game is *Name that Tune* where the contestants try to recognise a tune from as few notes as possible. Similar and more elaborate versions can be produced using electronic synthesisers. For example, there is great pleasure to be had from being able to identify bird songs and exercises based on them should prove very enjoyable for many.

(4) The importance of exercises that demand quick motor responses to sensory stimuli, i.e. sharp reaction times, was emphasised earlier. Francis Galton, the 19th century scientist and cousin of Charles Darwin predicted that more intelligent humans would respond more quickly to simple sensory stimuli compared to the less intelligent. This prediction has quite recently been verified in the laboratory.

A series of experiments in recent years at Edinburgh University, and also at the Institute of Psychiatry in London have found that the greater a person's IQ, the less time the individual takes to respond (by pressing a button) to simple stimuli such as a flashing light.

Leaving aside the notion of IQ, which is subject to controversy, we take it as self evident that being able to respond quickly to sensory stimuli is an indicator of health and that exercises that improve reaction times are beneficial.

Ball games such as squash and table tennis make demands on reaction times but they involve visual stimuli only and provide no accurate information on the quality of reaction. The computer can be used to design more complex reaction tasks involving a mixture of visual and aural stimuli and possibly others.

Despite their limitations, the games already available on microcomputers are of considerable value in this context. There are many persons whose training only includes jogging and weight training, activities that make little demand on the sharpness of reactions. Such persons will undoubtedly benefit by adding computer games to their programme. Computer games are particularly recommended for those over the age of fifty. No establishment that cares for the health of older persons should be without them.

Unfortunately, present day computer games rely on visual cues only. To exercise hearing we need games that incorporate aural cues. For example, we can imagine games where success comes from being able to recognise sounds at slightly different frequencies, or from being able to focus on a single sound in a mixture of other sounds, etc. What is needed of course is entirely new purpose-designed equipment that can engage the full range of sensory and motor activity.

Other senses

We chose to discuss the sense of hearing because it is frequently abused and the easiest one to cater for without very much specialised equipment. The central message, however, is applicable quite generally. All the senses can be developed to a far greater acuity and far better preserved with age than is the case today. Their functioning affects our health and vigour in myriads of ways. With computerised equipment it should be possible to exercise them efficently and to keep an eye on any signs of deterioration.

Like hearing, the extra equipment needed for the eyes would be minimal. The computer can readily produce shapes, characters of varying sizes and millions of colours of varying brightness and hues. It can switch information on and off at any rate that is likely to be needed. By attaching several monitors both the short- and long- distance visions could be exercised and the eyes made to interact with near and far objects and so on. With special equipment worn on a helmet three dimensional effects can be produced ad so on. Speed reading and comprehension are obvious examples of activities that could be combined with exercises that aim purely to move the eyes and test their sensitivity.

More specialist equipment would be demanded to exercise the kinesthetic sense (the sense of balance), e.g. a pressure sensitive platform that can, under the control of the computer, be made to swivel and tilt. The kind of activity we have in mind should become clear from the following example.

A game has been invented by a group of mechanical engineers from University College London for retraining the sense of balance of stroke patients. Many such persons suffer extreme unsteadiness on their feet and suffer damaging falls. Traditional physiotherapy methods of retraining are slow and lack the elements of novelty and fun.

To play the game the patient stands on a pressure sensitive platform which is connected to a TV screen. The patient controls the position of a cross on the screen through shifting his weight from foot to foot and also from heel to toe. Through this manoeuvre the patients tries to hit a series of targets and score points. Clearly, there is no limit to the variety and complexity of games that can be invented along these lines and such equipment would be of use generally in the fight against ageing.

One underdeveloped area that could be opened up in a radically new way through exploiting the computer has to do with the sense of touch.

Touch is the most ancient of senses in the evolution of the nervous system. It is through touching in the first instance that other senses have evolved and for this reason it has been referred to as 'the mother of senses'. We share this sense with all other animals, no matter how far down the evolutionary ladder. The whole of our skin is an organ of touch. Phrases such as 'being touched', 'being touchy', 'being in touch' express our awareness of this significance. Touching affects our health in all sorts of profound ways. For example, one recent finding is that stroking of pets is therapeutic for heart patients.

To exercise the sense of touch it would be necessary to wear electronically wired pads next to the skin which would produce computer driven sensations. The subject would learn to read these faint sensations in the way that a blind person learns to read braille, only a much broader skin surface could be utilised. To convince the reader that what is being suggested here is sensible and potentially of great value we shall hear from someone who has developed her sense of touch to a high level.

The author has been fortunate to have corresponded with Carolyn James, who lives in Scotland. She is blind yet she paints beautiful landscapes! She has developed her sense of touch to such a degree that she has not only overcome the limitations of being sightless but has positively come to rejoice in the discovery of heightened awareness that her lack of vision has brought to her.

Describing her deployment of touch, she wrote in a letter to the author, " If I want to really experience the atmosphere and the physical layout of a place, then I use every part of my body that I can decently use! For instance, on the beach I consciously use not only my toes and soles of my feet to find out the textures of what I am walking on, but I use the sensory nerves in my legs to become conscious of the wind, sand, water etc. I use my arms and hands in the same way, and my face. Funnily enough I find my cheeks are ultra-sensitive to the air.... When my nervous system is stimulated like this I then feel a physical change over my entire body. Quite quickly I feel a glowing sensation but an extreme one. I have ascertained that my skin does not change colour but this glowing goes right through every inch of my body both internally and externally. When I feel it reach the back of my neck, for it always begins in my toes, then mentally I feel light-headed. I feel as if there is a terrific space between my toes on the ground and my head. I am only 5'6" and my head could be 8' off the ground! It is a very real physical sensation, and one that I enjoy experiencing. At the same time emotionally I feel a complete calm internally and a great sense of being at one with my surroundings where I am not merely an onlooker". Near the end of letter she asks "Why can't the sighted people appreciate their world to this degree?"

Carolyn James and others like her exemplify what should be obvious. Our nervous system is our reality and the more acutely we learn to detect the signals that impinge on our nerve endings the more vivid becomes our reality. The more sensitively we can learn to touch, to smell, to taste, to hear, to see and to feel the temperature, the more vividly alive we can become. Although motivated by different aspirations, aspects of mysticism and meditation have simply been directed towards the discovery of heightened pleasure in awarenes as described so eloquently by Carolyn James. This has been achieved through exercises that focus concentrated attention on minutely isolated signals. Simone Weil the French mystic proclaimed, "Absolute attention is prayer", and one can understand why she said that.

The computer offers a more efficient route to what has previously been attained only laboriously. It would be relatively easy to make effective use of the computer to promote the sense of touch. This is so because highly sensitive tactile sensors, vastly more sensitive compared to human finger tips, are quite commonly in use in industrial applications, e.g. for handling fragile objects. This is one area where the sensitivity of machines far excels those of the human counterparts.

Apart from learning to touch sensitively there is the fundamental need to be touched and stroked rhythmically. Grooming and other forms of touch stimulation, such as licking, are widespread forms of behaviour throughout the animal world and they serve the needs of basic biological functions. For example, in many species, the touch stimulation of the genital areas is essential for the new born to learn the action of waste elimination. When such animals are reared without the presence of the mother then her licking action has to be simulated through stroking with a soft moist cloth. Without this the young die.

All ancient human cultures have extensively used touching to promote health. Hippocrates, the father of Western medicine stated "The physician must be experienced in many things but assuredly also in rubbing". Ayurveda, the great Sanskrit Classic on health advised the seeker after health to "rise early, bathe, clean the mouth, rub the body with oil and submit to friction massage before exercising". Annointing and laying on of hands has been a natural method for healing everywhere. Much of physiotherapy today continues to rely on nothing other than skilled rubbing.

Clearly the action of rubbing need have no emotional content to be pleasurable and therapeutic but there are obvious problems in finding humans to have oneself rubbed in this way. Not many are skilled and those that are, are costly. Humans get tired, they can make us feel self conscious, they expect us to rub them back and so on.

Intelligent robots that could give a range of skilled massage to order should prove a great boon to overcome these problems. This would not be all that a novel invention. Rich Romans, at the height of their Empire, spent hours lying around being massaged with perfumed oils by their dumb and castrated slaves. Their great orator statesman Cicero proclaimed that he owed his health as much to his anointer as to his physician. A computerised version of the annointer would go a long way towards banishing the billions of sleeping pills and anti-depressants that are currently prescribed and have nasty side effects. It could be a very effective weapon in the fight against stress.

The sensory environment

Health can only be discussed sensibly in the context of environments. Senses exist in environments and the sensory environment affects our body, mood thoughts and behaviour in a variety of profound ways. What we hear, what we see, what we touch, what we smell, in our environment all affects our functioning.

If laboratory animals are reared under differently coloured lights then the organs of their bodies grow at different rates. It has been found that a patient who has had his gall bladder removed needs more and stronger doses of analgesic, a longer hospital stay and more nursing if he has only a brick wall to look at , compared to a similar patient who can see trees and greenery. In 1971 Martha McClintock discovered that women who lived together in dormitaries tended to menstruate at the same time and later this effect was traced to being triggered through smell. Studies have shown that background music can help improve productivity and concentration. These are just a few examples of the continuous interactions between the sensory environment and our physiology.

The computer should be used to control the quality of our personal sensory environment and to regulate it intelligently. We could, for example, make more intelligent use of sounds in our everyday environment, particularly our work environment. Sounds can soothe and comfort, they can excite, they can help us concentrate, they can lull us to sleep. We now have the facility to make an unlimited range of sound available to affect our wellbeing.

Again the computer can cater for special requirements. For example, it has been found recently that bright light in measured doses can reset the internal body clocks of travellers suffering from jet lag. The computer serving the needs of a shift worker or the needs of someone who suffers from insomnia or Winter depressions could provide measured doses of bright light in their environments.

The computer can also act as a watch dog against the pollution of our sensory environments. Consider the case of noise. In addition to impairment of hearing, sustained experience of loud noise leads to difficulty in speech communication, lack of concentration, sleeplessness and of course annoyance. These factors can combine to lead to all sorts of other health problems. Reports have shown, for example, that areas affected by aircraft noise have far greater admissions to mental hospitals than average. There are also findings which point to more subtle connections between hearing centres and other control mechanisms in the brain. For example, it has been found that asthmatics can hear more high pitched sound than is normal.

A computerised watch over our sound environment would be valuable because we ourselves often fail to notice the build-up of dangerous noise. We can switch off (habituate) at a conscious level and continue to suffer damage. Apart from obvious sources such as planes, motorways, building construction and so on, which can introduce new noise, dangerous noise can also be introduced from some very simple household sources. Typically, an extractor fan may start emitting a high frequency sound which we fail to notice after a while. Even rural environments are not necessarily free from noise hazard. Bulldozers, farm machinery, chain saws, milking equipment and squealing pigs have all been implicated in noise-induced hearing defects.

Studies have shown that individuals differ substantially in their tolerance as well as vulnerability to sound. Thus social legislation may not be adequate for our personal needs. With computerised equipment we ourselves can decide the levels at which we should receive a warning.

Computers for the training of the imagination

Survival is only possible through being able to respond to the ever-changing significances implicit in the environment (including the body's internal environment). For this purpose the brain constantly monitors the environment at conscious as well as unconscious levels and adjusts metabolism accordingly.

If the external environment is perceived as being cold we start shivering. If the blood temperature rises by even a fraction of a degree then thousands of sweat glands go to work. If we see a police car we become nervous and tense. If we receive some unexpected good news then suddenly our jadedness disappears and we are exhilarated. We can picture the activity of the brain as comprising the following perpetual feedback loop:

Repeat until dead the following two steps:

(1) Use sensory apparatus and imagination to interpret current events in the environment (including the internal environment).

(2) Produce appropriate physiological changes.

The important point to appreciate is that our imagination is constantly involved in determining our future functioning. The benefits of pills, potions, diets, exercise, rituals, other treatments and events are all subject in varying degrees to what goes on in the imagination. This principle is no more weird, uncanny or supernatural than any other facet of reality, say the existence of electrons. It is simply a physiological property arising from electro-chemical events in the brain.

Before the advent of scientific medicine, spells, charms and rituals which relied entirely on imagination were the central methods available to humans to exercise control over physiological processes. Voodoo priests, shamans, witch doctors and others relied universally on the patients's powers of imagination to heal, to overcome fears, to build self esteem and so on. "Wen, wen, little wen, May you become as small as a linseed grain, and much smaller than the hipbone of an itchmate, and may you become so small that you become nothing" is a thousand-year-old Anglo-Saxon spell for curing boils. No doubt it worked for exactly the same reason that goat's testicles, sow's vulvae, crocodile's teeth and the right side of an elephant's trunk have all succeeded as potent aphrodisiacs in the past (see *Aphrodisiacs: The Science and the Myth* by Peter Taberner, Croom Helm).

Perhaps the observations of some aborigine tribes in northern Australia show most dramatically how potent can be the effects of the imagination. Here the chiefs have exercised the power to bring about the death of a tribesman within a specified period, e.g. within two days, merely by letting the victim know that he will die within that period.

A great deal of controlled scientific data on the influence of the imagination in determining the benefits of therapies has become available in recent years through studies involving placebos. Placebos contain no active ingredients (typically, they are coloured pills made out of flour and sugar) but in thousands of recorded cases have been found to be highly effective in producing the 'expected' medicinal effects. In some cases they have turned out to be even more effective than the actual medication and scholarly papers in learned medical journals have pleaded for much greater use of placebos in medicine to reduce costs and minimise the harmful side effects of real drugs.

Undoubtedly, the greatest health and fitness skill the individual needs is the facility to trigger day-to-day actions based on positive interpretations of the state of the world outside and the personal bodily states within. The writer and psychotherapist Sidney Jourard observed, "A person lives as long as he experiences his life as having meaning and value and as long as he has something to live for. As soon as meaning, value and hope vanish from a person's life, he begins to stop living; he begins to die". Meaning, value and hope are created through the interpretations we place on the world and on ourselves which in turn are the products of our imagination. Thus the primary health skills humans need have not to do with jogging or eating granary bread, rather they have to do with the construction of a positive imagination.

From the masses of grumbling that are heard everywhere one can easily conclude that the primary health skills are in very short supply indeed. Despite all that science, technology and rationality have done to transform the world and despite the unprecedented scale on which opportunities for self-fulfilment have become available, most humans live overwhelmingly with the perception that the state of the world has actually got worse.

Positive thinking, which should more accurately be called 'positive imagining', is often paid lip service to but no systematic or workable training of any sort is prescribed to develop it. It remains an attribute stumbled upon by genetic and environmental luck rather than something constructed by design and insight.

The "look good feel good" recipes suggest, sometimes explicitly and always implicitly, that fitness and muscle development necessarily lead to a positive view of life but this is not a fact. Very often the pursuit of fitness and concern for external form leads to a heightening of neurosis and dissatisfaction with self, factors which actually unleash the very processes they are supposed to prevent. Under the influence of this falsehood, the British Penal system, typically, has tried in recent years to cure young thugs through prescribing intensive fitness programmes involving weight training. P.E. and so on. These have proved abject failures. One only has to witness the antics of fit football hooligans and super fit tennis stars on TV to be forced to conclude that highly developed muscles can indeed exist with puny and self-destructive emotions. Equally, one only has to recall the muscular stature of someone like Mahatma Gandhi to be instantly convinced that a highly positive world view can thrive in a frail collection of skin and bones.

The health culture can make no significant advance unless it can offer methods for developing a positive imagination together with the usual muscle-based activities. Apart from its role in healthful day-to-day functioning, a positive imagination is needed for the overcoming of pain and stress which most of us need to do at some time or the other. It is essential for creativity and for the greater fulfilment of our potential. Indeed whatever humans desire, be it success, money, sex, creativity or anything else, imagination is the key ingredient. It is this attribute that gives humans their power over all other animals and until the gym can cater for this need it will essentially be serving very limited needs.

Before we discuss how the computer can be used for developing the imagination, we shall look at some examples of the way the powers of the imagination have been used deliberately to improve performance and combat disease. These examples are meant to make the case for finding the time to exercise the imagination.

Imaging

By "imaging" we mean the deliberate use of mental images to induce body processes. In some oriental cultures, such as yoga, imaging-type practices have been cultivated under the broad umbrella of meditation for a very long time. There are many well documented and authenticated records of extraordinary control over physiological functioning. The deliberate use in imaging in Western sport and medicine is, however, fairly recent though growing rapidly.

One of the first scientific investigations of the effect of imaging on performance in sport was carried out in Australia by Alan Richardson in the 1950's. He charted the improvement of throwing skill in three groups of basketball players. One group was set to practice twenty minutes of basketball throws in the gym. The second group spent the same amount of time only imagining going through the same exercises. The third group formed a control group and did no throwing exercises. Richardson discovered, that on average the group that had only done imaging exercises had improved their skill by the same amount as the group that had actually practiced in the gym.

Since then the use of imaging in sport has grown enormously and is now becoming a vital part of the coaching of top sportsmen and women, though it goes under the nonsensical name of "mind-over-matter". Some very famous champions and coaches have proclaimed this kind of training to be the secret of their success. For example, Lee Evans, who set a spectacular world record for the 400 metre dash in 1968, practiced imaging for several years before the actual event under the direction of his coach Bud Winter. Evans, it has been described, imagined every stride of the whole race and rehearsed every emotion that would be involved in the future event of winning.

A similar mental imagery based technique called *The Inner Game* has been widely promoted recently by Timothy Gallway and has attracted many famous persons as converts. Typically, in the Inner Game training for tennis or golf, the player is taught to practice, at first only in the imagination, the hitting of the ball repeatedly at the desired target. After this imagined practice the player then proceeds to perform the real actions. It is emphasised that the real playing should be done without trying very hard at the conscious level and trusting that right actions would surface automatically.

Imaging is also being utilised in a wide spectrum of settings in medicine. For example, it has been used to facilitate painless childbirth, to lower blood pressure in hypertensive patients and as an adjunct therapy in the treatment of cancer. Carl Simonton and Stephanie Matthews-Simonton, the world famous husband and wife team from the Cancer Counselling and Research Center in Dallas USA, have demonstrated that imaging can shrink and sometimes even eliminate the deadliest of cancers (see *Getting Well Again*, Bantam Books 1981) .

Some dramatic successes of imaging have been reported even in the fight against Aids. For example, in September 1985, the Aids Project of Los Angeles, the world's largest Aids organisation, sponsored Louie Nassaney for a Superman competition. Despite having contracted Aids and despite having succumbed to severe diarrhoea, headaches, hallucinations, fevers, weight loss and other debilitating symptoms he had managed to transform himself into being a fighting fit specimen and a champion body builder. Nassaney's case history was reported as follows.

In 1982 he had developed a lump on his leg which had been diagnosed as Kaposi's sarcoma, the form of skin cancer associated with Aids. At first he had received Interferon treatment but his condition had deteriorated rapidly. In early 1984 Nassaney had decided to come off the drugs and had taken matters into his own hands. He then turned to imaging and invented an exercise which involved imagining that the cancerous skin on his leg was a pencil mark which was being erased. After six months of this exercise, the cancerous bump on his leg apparently began to flatten out and then faded away altogether.

Nassaney then employed the same method to boost his T-cell count which had depleted drastically. As is well known now, it is this depletion that renders the immune system of Aids sufferers ineffective. He imagined that his T-cells were like little white rabbits that were breeding prolifically like other rabbits. It was documented that by the end of 1985 Nassaney's T-Cell count had reached almost normal. A number of similar, apparently well checked and authenticated, cases have been reported in the press.

A rational approach to the workings of the imagination

At present the fruits of the imagination in creating and maintaining positive expectations are mostly enjoyed by the credulous. "When travelling, I wear a holy medallion on my left wrist and a diamond cross on my right to save me from accidents. Both have been blessed", so wrote Miss Barbara Cartland, one of the doyens of mass health culture who recommends honey and buckets full of vitamins.

The reason why the credulous are mostly the beneficiaries is that the imagination is thought of in terms of the mind rather than in terms of the brain, i.e. in terms of magic rather than mechanism. Historically, the physiological and psychological effects of the imagination have been explained in terms of religion and magic. For this reason the subject continues to give rise to fears and feelings of uneasiness. The effects of imaging, for example, are always presented under the irrational heading of 'mind-over-matter' and generously sprinkled with words such as 'mysterious', 'miraculous', 'infinite' and so on. References to Buddhist temples, Catholic Stigmatics and Tibetan Lamas are usually followed by allusions to metal-bending, telepathy, precognition and so on. Instead of allowing any rational insights which may lead to procedures of practical value the whole subject is made to evaporate into a mystifying cloud of mumbo-jumbo.

To get rid of these weird associations and to develop the subject within a rational framework the first requirement is that we should stop describing phenomena in terms of the vague and nebulous concept of the mind. It is a truism that if we cannot logically define a concept, we cannot give rational explanations to questions involving that concept. We should give and seek explanations in terms of the material brain and avoid invoking the insubstantial mind. We should think of all mental states as being related to real material electro-chemical events and take it as a normal function of the material brain to bring about physiological changes in response to meanings in our environment. The meanings could concern changes in temperature and sunlight and equally they could concern threats to our love life.

We must also place finite limits on our expectations. Whereas it is true that imagination can alter physiology in a spectular way it is false to conclude, as is done by the credulous mind-over-matter fans, that these processes can violate in any way the laws of physics or biology. They may be amazing but so is the switching on of a TV set and seeing a picture of an event sent by a space probe from millions of miles away.

Although it is true that at present our understanding of the detailed workings of the brain is very limited, it is obvious that the meaning our imagination places on events in our environment cause the brain to alter the electro-chemistry of our body. The smell of food makes us salivate; the picture of a naked young woman causes a man's pupils to dilate and so on. Gradually we are learning more and more about the material concomitants of mental states. For example, we now know that negative emotions such as despair cause the brain to release STH (Somatotrophic hormone, which is one of the hormones also released when the body is fighting an infection). We also know that imagining performing a motor action produces reduced but similar electrical activity in the appropriate muscles.

Developing the imagination for day to day health

Our object now is to explain in rational terms how the imagination can be exercised deliberately for the creation of health. First we shall elucidate that which is of value for everyone. Later we shall look at more demanding requirements for those who would aspire to achieve more than the average individual.

The first insight one needs concerns the importance of language. Words and images determine our consciousness. The words we use generate images. Our language, or the words we use, constitute our perspective on external reality as well as on ourselves. Our capacity for self-awareness springs from our language. Some philosophers and thinkers have argued that consciousness is not merely a consequence of language, *IT IS* language (see, for example *Ancestral voices; Language and the Evolution of Human Consciousness* by C.G. Smith, Prentice Hall).

Leaving aside the philosophical issues concerning the nature of consciousness, it is an irrefutable fact that all of us are continuously engaged in silent internal monologues. "... must phone the insurance company... this is terrible... let's finish this chapter... I did enjoy that Pizza... give jogging a miss this evening..." etc. are typical silent monologues that reverberate perpetually in our brain. This silent monologue, more than any other attribute, characterises our consciousness and also determines what we say to others. Our interpretation of the world and of our own place in it is determined by this monologue. Thus whether we see the world as a place of beauty and hope or of despair and ugliness is determined at the root by the nature of the words we use in conducting this internal monologue.

We state the following fundamental principle: **We transform our perspective over external reality and over ourselves when we tranform what we say to ourselves and to others.**

To appreciate how profoundly human perspective and control on events is determined by the language they use consider the last words of Bishop Hugh Latimer, uttered in 1555 on his way to being burnt alive for heresy. He is recorded to have said, "Be of good comfort,..and play the man. We shall this day light such a candle by God's grace in England as I trust shall never be put out".

By choosing to use the right words human imagination can place positive interpretations on even the most horrendous circumstances. "Drag your thoughts away from your troubles-by the ears, by the heels, or any other way you can manage it. It is the healthiest thing a body can do", advised Mark Twain. We can manage the task if we develop the skill to control what we tell ourselves about our situation.

The language patterns we use to interpret events are at present determined randomly. The health culture so far has no clear insight into promoting the use of language for triggering healthy emotional responses. Some people are naturally gifted with healthful language patterns. The famous French dancer and singer Mistinguett when asked by a journalist whether a woman's sexual appetite declined with age replied, "How should I know, I'm only seventy". Most persons, however, are inclined to employ language to interpret events in a way that causes unnecessary damage to themselves. Later we shall see how the computer can be used to eradicate this major source of loss of vigour and vitality.

Developing the imagination for extraordinary powers

A person with a high degree of control over his imagination can enjoy all sorts of extraordinary powers over circumstances. Control over body processes are particularly of interest to us here. To identify clearly for the reader what is involved in the exercise of such powers we shall use a case study. It is taken from the biography of the famous stage performer and hypnotist Romark by Ursula Markham (*Hypno-think,* Thorsons). Romark once suffered a stroke and was hospitalised. This is how he described an incident which took place during that period.

'When I was in hospital after the stroke they wanted me to use a bedpan, but I didn't like the idea. I decided to use the toilet in the normal way... I knew for a fact that I was paralysed and that I couldn't walk. But I forced myself to imagine that I could walk as far as the toilet. I pictured myself walking as far as the toilet, and I convinced myself that I had, in fact, walked to the toilet.

I did this step by step - a laborious process. I didn't just imagine in general terms that I got up and went to the toilet. I pictured in my mind's eye every single detail - every move involved in the whole trip... I hadn't actually done it yet, so the action I contemplated - and which I saw clearly in my mind - still lay in the future.

Finally, I convinced myself - still within my imagination - that I had actually made the trip to the toilet and returned to my hospital bed. At that point I got out of bed, walked to the toilet and came back to bed once more without any conscious effort. The nurses, of course, were amazed.'

The crux of the matter in the above description is contained in the following key phrases:

(i) **I did this step by step ... I didn't just imagine in general terms that I got up and went to the toilet. I pictured in my mind's eye every single detail - every move involved in the whole trip.**

(ii) **Finally, I convinced myself - still within my imagination - that I had actually made the trip ... and came back to bed once more without any conscious effort.**

To be able to exercise the sort extraordinary powers over our circumstances that are referred to as mind-over-matter we essentially need two skills. Firstly we need the skill to imagine in great detail.

Going back to Richardson, to whom we referred earlier, he found that the improvement in basketball throwing that took place purely through imagined practice depended very much on the range of the subject's imagination. Those who could imagine the moving ball did better than those who could only imagine the static court and the basket. Those who could imagine the sounds associated with the bouncing ball did better than those who could not; those who could also imagine the tactile feeling of the ball thumping the hand at each bounce did even better and so on.

Secondly we need the skill to convince ourselves (for short periods) that an event has taken place in the real world which has actually happened only in the imagination. The two skills we have identified are of course not unconnected. Clearly, the more vividly an event is imagined the greater is the conviction produced of it being real. The combination of a vivid imagination with conviction or faith is the font of all those events that have been described as being magical and miraculous. It is through the deliberate cultivation of these skills that some humans, e.g. some adepts of meditation, have managed to 're-wire' their nervous system and vastly extend their potential.

It should now be possible to see clearly that what is needed is a tool that can help us develop our facility to imagine in great detail and with appropriate feelings. We need to imagine the full spectrum of sensory inputs - the shapes, the colours, the sounds, the smells, the tastes and the tactile feelings. The tool should be be able to create convincing artifical realities. Undoubtedly the computer, with suitable additions, is the most powerful tool that can be used for this purpose and in this way offers revolutionary possibilities for humans to learn to control their health.

To make a radical and lasting change in our situation and behaviour demands persistence. The American Poetess Ella Wheeler Wilcox said, "Man is what he thinks. Not what he says, reads or hears. By persistent thinking you can undo any condition which exists. You can free yourself from any chains, whether of poverty, sin, ill health, unhappiness or fear". It would have been more accurate of course if she had used the phrase "persistent imagining", however, she does spell out the need for persistence.

The first reason why the computer is an appropriate tool is that with its help it becomes easy to exercise persistence. Most people never get far with positive imagining because they are only able to keep it up for a few days. The effort to keep going demands large amounts of motivation and will power. Once the computer has been programmed it can keep going through repeat performances as long as we like.

We shall later give an example program which demands only five minutes or so of regular interaction and takes the reader through a structured sequence of exercises. The same exercises could be done without the computer but would demand much greater motivation.

For the purposes of developing powers of visualising shapes, the role of the computer is very easy to grasp. Everyone is aware that the computer can readily produce images of all sorts. It is being used by engineers for designing real objects as well as by artists for creating images that arouse feelings.

Although the feeling of true three-dimensonality produced by conventional equipment is rather limited, the computer has been shown to be a powerful tool for learning to visualise shapes in 3-D and is being used for this purpose in the training of designers in Computer Aided Design. This facility is at a surprisingly high premium universally and research has shown that even such professionals as crystallographers and architects whose work involves much 3-D visualisation experience great difficulty. Research has also shown that with suitable exercises remarkable improvements in 3-D visualisation can be achieved [see *3D Visualisation* by R.D. Parslow in Eurographics 82 published by North Holland].

New equipment now being developed in the USA and Britain will make the computer a far more powerful tool for these purposes. For example, Dr. John

Waldern of Loughborough University in U.K. has designed a helmet which carries a stereoscopic optical system. The wearer of the helmet experiences computer-produced graphics as if they were the three-dimensional reality in which he existed. This kind of equipment will soon be available for arcade-type game playing and would be very suitable for adaptation to imagination training.

Finally, let us now show how every individual might gain enormous benefits from a computerised version of meditation. Let us consider some of the personal attributes that go with a healthy and positive existence. Most will agree that we need a temperament that reinforces strengths and successes and minimises weaknesses and failures. They will also agree that we need to cultivate real skills of effectiveness. Clear goals, powers of concentration and memory, resilience in the face of problems, good management of time and energy and the skill to cooperate with suitable partners are some examples of such skills.

To create these skills we need a tool that offers intelligence as well as profound images. The tool should allow us to experience regularly and vividly the illusion of being in possession of such skills and attributes as we desire. It should also help us carry that illusion into reality. Typically, to develop clarity of purpose as a living health skill the tool should conjure up for us a whole range of scenarios which would show us performing in just such a way and help us act out these scenarios in our imagination. It should then help us create clarity of purpose. Computerised equipment driven by intelligent software can provide the kind of tool that meets the bill.

We conclude this chapter by offering the reader a simple program for computerised imagination training that requires no special equipment. The programme runs in what the author calls the Socratic mode. It merely asks a series of loaded questions and invites responses. These questions and suggestions force the reader to think, feel and imagine along certain lines that have been carefully chosen.

Before executing the program the subject should relax deeply and rapidly, a task in which the computer could also assist. Ideally the program should execute automatically each day when the machine is switched on first. This is a major benefit offered by the computer since it obviates the need for will power. The program merely outputs the following series of statements each time a key is pressed.

WHAT ARE YOUR DREAMS?
VISUALISE EACH DREAM VIVIDLY IN THE PRESENT.
RE-LIVE YOUR PAST SUCCESSES.
WHAT ARE YOUR PLANS? GIVE DATES.
WHAT PERSONAL QUALITIES DO YOU POSSESS?
MAKE PLANS FOR TODAY.
CHOOSE TODAY'S MAJOR ACCOMPLISHMENT.

Before we explain the logic behind these statements we would like to establish a very profound principle. The overall purpose of the computer program is not only to develop our capacity to imagine but also to transform what we say to ourselves. In the book *Journey to Ixtlan* by Carlos Castaneda, to make the negative and self-critical Carlos succeed, the wise don Juon tells him, "From now on, and for a period of eight days, I want you to lie to yourself. Instead of telling yourself the truth, that you are ugly and rotten and inadequate, you will tell yourself that you are completely the opposite". Don Juon was giving Carlos a very powerful piece of wisdom indeed which few humans understand or avail themselves of in any systematic way. Our program has the same purpose in mind as intended by don Juon. Let us explain it further.

WHAT ARE YOUR DREAMS ?

It was Oscar Wilde who said, "Don't part with your illusions. When they are gone you may still exist but you would have ceased to live". To be living and growing we have to have to keep on dreaming tenaciously with our eyes open.

The purpose of this question is to put the user in touch with his absolute authentic self everyday, something which few adults dare to do. The virtue of the computer is that the user can respond with complete honesty and without any self consciousness. The user can dream epic dreams without fear of being made to appear foolish.

As use continues, the user is expected to refine his dreams and add more and more flesh and bones to them. Typically he might go from saying, "I want to write a best seller", to "I want to write a best seller on health", to "I want to write a best seller on health that shows how computers can be used to revolutionise health" and so on.

Finally, it should be appreciated that the very act of specifying something in detail is itself a solution. The act of specifying our dreams in great detail will, with high probability, lead to insight on how to satisfy them. In any case, even if the mere specification is not by itself sufficient, it is surely a necessary requirement. As the famous song goes, "You gotta hava dream. If you donhava dream ..then how ya gonna maka dream come true?"

VISUALISE EACH DREAM IN THE PRESENT

A major trick in making dreams come true is to imagine for short periods that the dream has already been fulfilled. Many persons have stumbled on it. Joe Karbo, the author of *"The lazy Man's Way to Riches "* claimed to have made himself a multi-millionaire using just this trick. Joe Karbo, who died a few years ago, but whose book is still making a fortune, proclaimed that absolutely anyone could have absolutely anything they wanted by this method.

We do not understand enough about the brain to be able to explain the exact mechanism behind this process, but most probably through experiencing the fulfillment of our dreams for short periods, unconscious inhibitory behaviour patterns which keep us from grasping the opportunities in our environment are damped out. Also, it is quite likely that we unconsciously begin to communicate to others the kind of signals that cause them to cooperate in the fulfilment of our dreams.

This is a stage where specialised equipment would be appropriate to help the user imagine the fulfillment of his dreams in the present.

RE-LIVE YOUR PAST SUCCESSES
Most people spend their time focussing only on their flaws and failures. Analysis of failure may be useful in small doses but if the memories of success are blotted out then the whole thing becomes destructive. Recalling experience of past success is highly therapeutic. It is health giving. It is an act of friendship towards oneself and an encouragement to oneself to grow.

WHAT ARE YOUR PLANS?
This question is meant to force the user to set clear short -and-long term goals, to make definite intelligible plans and to manage time. The computer is an ideal tool for constructing, refining and displaying plans. It can show us the overview of our goals as well as the details. It can show us where we are and where we are planning to be. Ideally one would like a computerised response to this question. By pressing some special key at this stage the computer should go into DISPLAY/ CREATE PLANS MODE and should show us our plans as well as allow us to make changes if we desire.

In the absence of any elaborate software, the user can respond from a written list which will show life goals and also contain markers for all the major things that the user is intending to achieve in the near future - "by September 15th I will complete writing Chapter 5. In early December I will take a course in horse riding", etc.

WHAT PERSONAL QUALITIES DO YOU POSSESS ?
The logic behind this question was explained earlier. It is intended to make the user verbalise positively about himself.

The user is expected to use potent words to describe the qualities which he regards as most worthy. It is not our intention to tell the reader the exact qualities he should choose, but self-confidence, authenticity, clear goals, good management of time and energy, social skills, capacity for relaxation, service to others, a balanced programme of fitness and nutrition are examples of the kind of skills that need to be cultivated for overall health. We will give two examples of the kind of words that might be used in response to this question. It must be emphasised that the user must choose his own set of words. Further, since the nervous system habituates, words loose their power and from time to time the responses should be recouched. Again, appropriate intelligent software could be made available to help construct powerful sets of words.

SELF CONFIDENCE: "I never question my potential. I have unflinching faith in myself. I stand in awe of my possibilities. I am resolute, capable and self assured. I refuse to withdraw. I refuse to be beaten. I have a stubborn determination that thrives on challenges".

SERVICE TO OTHERS: "I am a gifted giver of life to others. Whosoever knows me receives the gift of significance, of wonder, of fascination. I encourage others to grow and fulfil their dreams.

MAKE PLANS FOR TODAY.

There may be days when it would be appropriate to do a random walk though life and make no plans at all. Such days are, for most people, only enjoyable if the rest of our days are managed efficiently and in keeping with our dreams and plans.

At this stage the user is expected to consult his diary (which with improved interface will be handled by the computer) and plan the day on a suitable form. The form should have headings for priority areas that reflect long-term aspirations and also for the usual day-to-day things such as phone calls, letters and errands.

CHOOSE TODAY'S MAJOR ACCOMPLISHMENT.

Success, it has been said, begets success. The object of this suggestion is to make the user experience success every day. After the day has been planned one activity should be marked as the day's key accomplishment. Come hell or high water the user should go all out to complete this task. After completing this task the user should allow himself a moment of satisfaction and a pat on the back. In this way the user can form the habit of success which has radical implications for long-term performance, health and preservation.

Closing Comments

In the early part of this century, the pioneer psychologist J. McKeen Cattell wrote, "We have in large measure explored the material world and subdued it to our uses; it is now our business to secure an equal increase in our knowledge of human nature and to apply it for our welfare".

Although our knowledge of human nature has greatly increased, relatively speaking, we have only employed the knowledge gained of the material world for our welfare. Before we can apply the knowledge gained of human nature we must adapt it to suit our unique personality by taking autonomous action. The computer is the best aid we possess for this purpose. The insignia of life is growth and transformation. The computer is a life tool because it can help each individual transform himself as he sees fit. We wish the reader life and happy transformation.

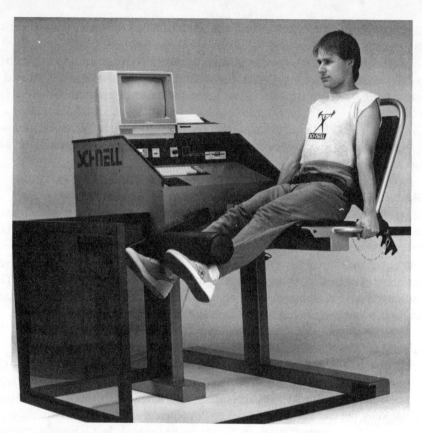

Fig 4.1. MODAR marketed by Schnell.

References & Suggestions for Further Reading

Brain-centredness: The satisfaction of human potential on a far greater scale than is the case today will only become possible when humans learn to think in terms of the brain. Today's thinking in health culture is muscle-centred, or stomach-centred or at best heart-and-lung-centred. These approaches are necessarily limited, fragmented and grossly out of focus. We have discovered that the brain of a creature is not simply a part of the creature, it is THE creature. The first set of references provide information about brain and behaviour.

1. Teyler, T.J., "A Primer of Psychobiology", W.H. Freeman, 1984. (*A good starting brief book on brain and behaviour for the general reader . Completely free of jargon , defines all technical terms.)*

2. Bloom, F.E., Lazerson, A. and Hofstadte, L., "Brain , Mind and Behaviour", W.H.Freeman 1985. (*An excellent and comprehensive book for the general reader. Particularly recommended for its 3-D diagrams*)

3. Changeux, J.P., " Neuronal Man: the biology of mind ", Pantheon , New York. 1985. (*Perhaps the most lucid guide on the subject of neurophysiology for the layman. The author brings a unified approach to explaining the brain and the 'mind' and relates mental acts to material correlates in the structures of the brain .)*

4. Campbell, H.J., "The Pleasure Areas", Methuen 1973 . (*One of the few books that set out to discuss very broad ethical problems directly in terms of neurophysiological structures . Very informative on the nature of the pleasure centres in the brain.)*

5. Springer, S. and Deutch, G., "Left Brain , Right Brain", W.H. Freeman 1985. (*A highly readable and fascinating account of our knowledge of the functions of the two halves of the brain. Dispels some of the over-simplified myths that have taken root in recent years on the division of functions between the two halves.*)

6. Klopf, A.H., " The Hedonistic Neuron ", Hemisphere, 1983 (*This is a fairly technical book but is highly original and is recommended to a mathematically educated reader. It ascribes purposive behaviour to the brain cell and shows, for example, how many of the gross observed features of learning and memory can then be predicted. The basic hypothesis is that neurons seek pleasure via electrical excitation. Behaviour of higher structures, including social structures, is then viewed as a consequence of cell behaviour at the lowest level.*)

7. Mueller, C.G., "Sensory Psychology", Prentice Hall, New Jersey, 1965. (*Excellent for basic information on sensory structure and psychology.*)

References below are on the powers of the imagination to alter physiology, performance and also external circumstances.

8. Richardson, A., "Mental Imagery", Springer, 1952 also Routledge and Keegan Paul, 1969. *(Richardson carried out early scientifically controlled experiments on the effects of mental imagery. This book describes his findings.)*

9. Playfair, G., "If this be Magic", Cape 1985. *(The book gives insight into the necessary and sufficient conditions for mind-over-matter magic to work. Has powerful practical implications.)*

10. Hill, N., "Think and Grow Rich", Wilshire Books, 1966. *(This is a classic book of its type on the so called positive thinking. Like all books of its kind it oversells the 'magic' of positive thinking. Nevertheless it offers extremely valuable insight.)*

11. Rivlan, R., "The Algorithmic Image", Microsoft Press, 1986. *(The book presents a very wide-ranging survey to show how computer graphics has aided in giant leaps of the imagination in the visual media in USA.)*

The greatest use of computers in trying to satisfy human potential has so far been in the education of the young and in particular the young handicapped. Some of the lessons learnt are highly relevant for extending human frontiers in general and for the combat of ageing. References below are on the use of computers in education.

12. Oshea, T. and Self, J., "Learning and Teaching with Computers", Harvester 1984. *(A wide ranging survey on the use of computers in the field.)*

13. Pappert, S., "Mind Storms", Harvester 1982. *(Pappert is a pioneer who has shown how computers can extend the learning potential of young children. Health Education desperately needs its own Pappert.)*

14. Goldenberg, E.P., "Special Technology for Special Children", University Park Press, Baltimore 1979. *(This is a review of computerised aids for handicapped children. Very great progress has been made in recent years in opening up the possibilities for such children through brain-centred approaches. Similar approaches are relevant in the combat of ageing.)*